Sound Advice

How to Help Your Child with SPD, Autism and ADHD from the Inside Out

Robin C. Abbott, MS, OTR/L

Loving Healing Press
Ann Arbor, MI

Sound Advice: How to Help Your Child with SPD, Autism and ADHD from the Inside Out
Copyright © 2022 by Robin C. Abbott. All Rights Reserved

Learn more at www.booksoundadvice.com

ISBN 978-1-61599-676-6 paperback
ISBN 978-1-61599-677-3 hardcover
ISBN 978-1-61599-678-0 eBook

Published by
Loving Healing Press
5145 Pontiac Trail
Ann Arbor, MI 49105

www.LHPress.com   Tollfree 888-761-6268
info@LHPress.com   FAX 734-663-6861

Distributed by Ingram Book Group (USA/CAN/AU)

Contents

Table of Figures

Sidebars

Acknowledgements

This book is the effort of years of cogitation, revision and encouragement on the parts of so many people. As I'm sure is true with most authors, I'm concerned I will accidentally omit someone who was crucial in the creation of this volume. I hope they will forgive me. Foremost thanks to my first "kiddos", my children Ellie and Simon. Thanks for being my guinea pigs and all-around fantastic lab rats. I love you. Ellie, this book is clearer and more concise because of your talents in graphic design, you talented kid! Thanks to my husband, Chris, for thinking I'm so much awesomer than I really am. To Mom and Dad, Andrea and Ron Henry, thanks for the excellent grammatical awareness and love of books and writing.

I owe a debt of gratitude to Dr. Shelly Lane, for realizing that I'm terrible at research so I could put my energies elsewhere, and to the late Dr. Marie Anzalone, who said I was a "good writer"; I took that scant praise and turned it into a book. Special thanks to Dr. Susan Barry, who gave the horrible first draft a gracious look and said it was interesting enough to read.

Thanks to Katie Yancosek, my lifelong friend and cheerleader for being my book doula. Special thanks to Britta Conner for being an early reader and parent-perspective giver. The photos would never have happened without the generous involvement of Maggie Verdun and Shelly and James Chinn; thanks for your willingness! And a literary shout-out to Missy, Dan, Dustin, Pat and all the fabulous writers of Writers on the Avenue. You kept me going!

1 Children Are Not Short Grown-ups

Occupational therapists (OTs) are a funny bunch. No one really knows what we do. It's something of an inside joke among us. It's like being in a secret club that we desperately wish wasn't secret. When we do get a socially relevant shout-out, even if it's a silly or incorrect characterization like Matt Damon's character in *Downsizing*, we get a little over-excited. We geek out. When the *Today Show* did a piece several years ago on the OT who treated Al Roker's son, who is developmentally-delayed, well, we were tickled pink.

When watching the opening scene in the movie *Tully*, I perked right up when Charlize Theron uses the Wilbarger Sensory Therapeutic Brushing Protocol, an OT-developed technique, on her son. (Quick note: She's doing it wrong. It is not a how-to video). Later in the movie, Theron's character sounds completely defeated as she confides in her babysitter that no one could tell her *why* her son Jonah was so challenging; she didn't think therapy had been helpful. During the course of the story, Jonah gets kicked out of his school for his behaviors and has a melt-down in the bathroom of his new school because of the sound of the flushing toilet.

I had a very emotional reaction to the small story of Jonah. The movie was very good, by the way, but Jonah's story made me feel frustrated and angry and sad. I knew I could help Jonah. I could help his parents understand why he chose challenging behaviors and how to help him be more comfortable in the world. Why hadn't his therapist really helped this family?! Why hadn't anyone explained what was wrong with Jonah?! Why was I getting so upset? Jonah's family was fictional. Except they weren't. I recognized the love and concern Theron's character felt for her child, and the despair and frustration she felt because she couldn't help him. I have always thought of my work with children as making the road of parenting smoother for families. As a mother, I can think of no more important use of my time. For years, I have met versions of Jonah's family in my therapy practice. I know hundreds of Jonahs, and I've helped hundreds of Jonahs. I am even more frustrated and angry and sad for the families that come to me *after* having the same experience Jonah and his mother had.

One of my favorite things about working in this field is that, in giving families a new way to look at their child's behavior, it can free them from a lot of the guilt and frustration they can feel about their child being different from his or her peers. In the 1970s, occupational therapist A. Jean Ayres published *Sensory Integration and the Child*, a primary "bible" for a pediatric OT. She was among the first to articulate how children with learning disabilities process sensations differently and that therapy can increase awareness and processing of sensations to help children create adaptive responses to successfully interact with the world. This work was groundbreaking. It gave parents and educators a better understanding of the children they are trying to help. More importantly, therapy for sensory integration differences removed the stigma related to delayed learning and developmental disabilities. Ayres's ability to describe the internal world and struggles of the "clumsy" or "slow" child allowed for the discovery of the strengths of these children and how best to provide input in a way that made sense to them.

When viewed this way, a child's behavior is no longer a result of what a parent is doing wrong. It's not a parent's failure that they try seventeen things suggested by parenting magazines or well-meaning family and friends, and seem to constantly fail. Understanding the true root of a child's difficulties, even if the problem is not immediately "fixable" allows a parent to realize that their child is not behaving a certain way just to make them frustrated. This is not to say that behavioral, pharmacological and/or other sensory interventions for problem behaviors would not be effective. However, understanding the reason the problem occurred may lead to a different sequence of therapy, a different intervention, or no therapy at all. Understanding your child can help him understand himself, limit some of his frustration, and boost his self-esteem.

As I began my decade-plus of working with children with special needs, I struggled to understand why seemingly simple things for some children were so much more difficult for the children I saw in the clinic. Learning something new, adapting to small changes, or communicating simple ideas were seemingly impossible. In seeking answers, I wasn't just learning how to help children with challenges. I was learning what motivates us *all* to learn and develop. I was coming to understand that each person's brain might understand the same sensations in different ways and what made a person's behavior fall outside the range of "normal." Most gratifyingly, I learned how to help a child change the way they interpret their world, so that it is less frightening, more friendly and more instructive.

Parents, educators, and therapists can benefit from understanding how and why every human is motivated to learn. Not only can we better understand ourselves, but we can apply that knowledge to a child from a place of empathy and understanding. In this book, we will explore the development and function of the auditory and vestibular systems of the inner ear. My goal is to help you, the reader, understand how these systems impact daily behaviors and choices for all of us, and how the derailment of these systems can impact a child's learning and behavior.

Most of all, I want to offer hope. There *are* effective methods for changing the underlying neurology involved in these systems. Your child can participate more fluidly and functionally in their lives. With a better foundation of auditory and vestibular function, established through appropriate therapy, a child can be a more willing family member, a better learner at school, and a more communicative person—finally letting the amazing human they are shine for everyone. Understanding how your own brain developed to influence can help you understand the choices you have made; whether you are an introvert or an extrovert, or why you require a quiet or a noisy space to work efficiently, or why you love or hate rollercoasters.

From before birth, the vestibular system creates neural connections that help us understand our position in space and how we navigate through it. Our auditory system creates neural connections that help us understand the space in which we find ourselves, its size and shape, and the friends and foes within it. These two systems combine to create a kind of internal GPS that helps us interpret where we are, where we would like to go, and what information we need to get there. When our internal GPS breaks down, the result can be disorientation, anxiety, withdrawal from the world, and the over-activation of the neurological fight-or-flight response.

If the vestibular and auditory systems are not addressed adequately, therapy for a child's deficits will be less effective and more frustrating. Simply put, there is no work-around for effective vestibular and auditory therapy. Learning what these therapies look like will help you seek them out for your child. If the therapy your child is receiving doesn't seem to be making a difference to your family, that means it's not making a difference for your child. Please stop wasting your precious time, energy, and money. Use the information I share in this book to seek out therapy that will be as effective and efficient as possible.

Over several years, I learned how effective auditory and *regimented* vestibular therapy was in helping children with challenges, because I saw it working. As I made decisions about therapy with my clients based on the function of the vestibular and auditory systems, the children often made unexpected progress. These positive responses were often a more relaxed child, a more communicative child, a more successful child: improvements I couldn't account for any other way other than a focus on auditory and vestibular intervention.

This type of therapy, combined with therapy methods to address specific behavioral concerns, worked more quickly than anything else I had tried. I loved the stories parents would bring me about the new thing their child could do, or the thing they *stopped* doing, that made their family's lives smoother and happier, and made for a calmer, more loving home. Not only could their child perform the skills that we had been working on in therapy, but parents would also tell me of their child's new success in areas we *weren't* directly addressing in therapy. Parents were thrilled that their child could eat with utensils, or sleep through the night, or take a bath without a tantrum. But none of these things were necessarily skills we had been addressing through therapy. It seemed like magic.

My curiosity about why these therapies were so effective became something of an obsession. Courses for certification in these therapies introduced me to the theory on which they are based, and were instructive about *how* to perform the interventions. But I wanted to learn more about the neurological bases for the changes I was seeing, the *why* of how the brain works. I'm kind of a neurology geek. I read popular books on how the brain functions in my spare time. What I read in those books jibed well with what I was seeing in the clinic. But I had more questions than answers.

I delved into the academic research. And I found that scientists in many different fields were studying the theories on which vestibular and auditory interventions are based. Audiologists and sound engineers were studying how sound is processed in the brain, child development specialists were conducting experiments to discover how children learn and what can go wrong for special needs children, and neurologists were studying how movement is processed by the brain and what effect a malfunctioning vestibular system can have on behavior. Please be aware that I did not author any of the theories of human development that you'll encounter here. I am simply synthesizing what I have learned and what I have seen in working with hundreds of children and their families.

Over the years, I have given lectures on this information to other therapists (occupational, physical, and speech), educators and parents. In almost every situation, I see light-bulb moments of understanding that how we all develop, mentally, emotionally and physically, is impacted by auditory and vestibular function. When I present this information to other professionals, I often hear exasperation and frustration that they did not already know this information. Late in this book, I attempt to offer an explanation about this gap in professional knowledge. This book is my attempt to share what I have learned about positively affecting children's learning and behavior. I believe that when there are more people who truly understand how interactions with the physical world develop, there are more people to help children and families live their best and most successful life.

How to Use This Book

Because I took the time to write them, I'd like you to read all the words. However, you have a life. So, I suggest two ways to use this book.

For those of you with limited time (and isn't that everybody?), I recommend reading or skimming each chapter to give you an overview of the concepts. If you run into a new-to-you word or concept, and it is printed in **bold**, then it will be defined in the Glossary at the end of this book. Chances are you have never thought about how you interact with the world around you in quite this way. Spend some time figuring out what these concepts mean for you and how you perceive the world. The more you understand how the vestibular and auditory system interact with your conscious and unconscious mind, the more easily you can apply these concepts to the child you care about.

You may be concerned about specific behaviors and are looking for specific answers. While this is not designed to be that sort of book, I have created an index to specific behaviors at the back of this book, which will lead you to **bolded and underlined** text on the referred page. Read the area before and after the text (or the call-out box, if that's where the reference is). It may frame the difficulty your child is having in a new way or give you a new direction to work in. Additionally, you might review the Database Types in Chapter 9, to see if one of the categories best describes the child you are working with. There are case studies dispersed throughout and at the end of the Appendix, which might shed light on specific behaviors, or may be an insight into your child.

The second way to use this book is by taking more of a deep dive. I have used my experience with hundreds of children, distilled a few case studies, and presented the research that supports why I see the results I see clinically. Because the perspective is my own, and I treat every child who comes to my clinic with some form of auditory and vestibular therapy, you'll learn why I do this. Before you understand the "why", you may be curious about the "what." What does this type of therapy look like in practice? What should you be looking for in your own child's therapy? To satisfy your curiosity, I'll outline some methods and ideas here, but your understanding of why these methods help will form as you continue to read.

Regardless of how you choose to read this book, make sure you visit the "Caveats" section of Chapter 10, as those exceptions may refer to your child.

Vestibular Therapy

An effective clinic environment has equipment to move a child in multiple directions and varying speeds. There should be equipment to move her, independent of her motor participation, such a machine- or therapist-driven devices, swings or platforms. There should be opportunities for movements that are larger, stronger or more novel than those he can participate in elsewhere. If swinging on the swings at the playground were the intervention every child needed, then my clinic would not exist. There should be a variety of swings and a point from which they are mounted, fairly high off the ground and far from objects, so that big arcs of swinging, and sometimes crazy spinning, are possible. There should also be toys that allow a variety of movements that *are* under the child's control; like climbing walls, loft spaces to jump from, and ride-on toys. Once a child's brain has been alerted to sensations from their inner ears, the next step is to integrate that information into the way they move through the world, so I need things in my clinic that get them moving.

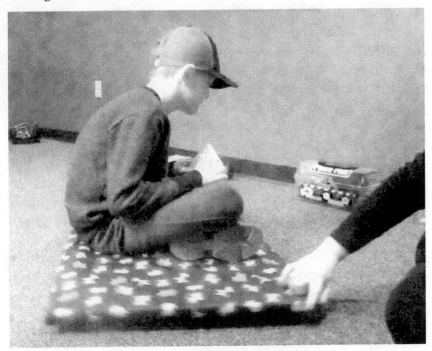

Fig. 1-1: A child seated on a rotary board

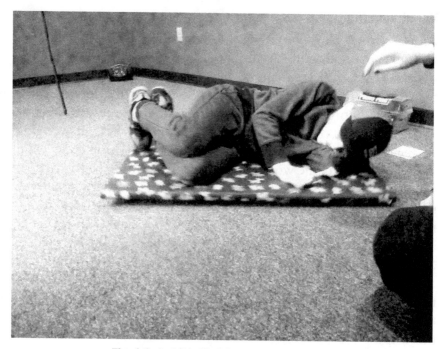

Fig. 1-2: A child side-lying on a rotary board.

In my clinic, I have several rotating platforms that are large enough for a child to lie down on their side, curled up. These platforms are used in a vestibular-ocular-motor program that I love, called Astronaut Training©. Astronaut Training is commercially available and easy to follow. I often assign it as daily at-home therapy for families, and I find that after a month of daily therapy, the child's vestibular system is much more functional and they can discontinue the program and move on.

The second element of appropriate vestibular therapy is a theoretically-driven sequence of types of movements. A therapist should be able to answer the questions, "What reaction are you expecting from a child when they participate in this movement? What change are you looking for from this movement? After they have incorporated this type of movement and have a functional response, what will you be asking them to do next?" Answers to these questions not only help a parent understand what the specific activity is for, but what progress will look like and how this moves a child toward their goal, whatever that may be.

Even during an evaluation, I receive clues from a child that tell me in what direction vestibular movement needs to progress. After meeting 20-month-old Amy, I spent the next ten-or-so minutes following her around the room, waiting to see what toys would engage her interest. While she aimlessly made her laps around the room, she parroted often-used phrases in her world, "Please", "Thank you" and "Amy", that had no bearing on what was actually occurring around her. I realized I would not be able to engage her while she was on the move, so I decided to put her in my net swing (see Fig. 1-3). I don't usually put a child in the net swing during an evaluation, but I was trying to save myself some energy. The net swing was a regular crowd-pleaser, so it seemed like a safe choice.

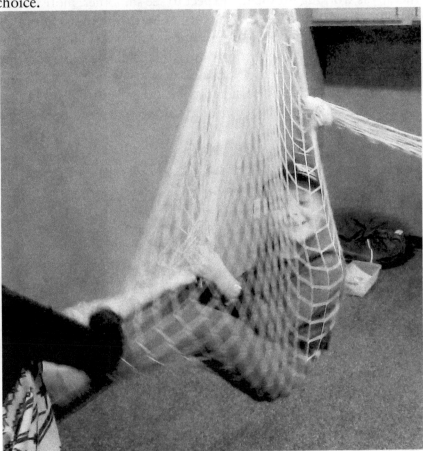

Fig. 1-3: Child engaged in big movement in the net swing.

After a few minutes of large swings, she looked straight at me with her big, brown eyes and said, "Hello." In reading this book, you'll learn *why* this type of movement helped Amy orient to her surroundings and interact more appropriately.

The final piece of effective vestibular therapy is incorporation. As a therapist, I should see hallmarks in a child's function that tell me that they are incorporating vestibular information into their movements and plans of action. One element of therapy in my clinic is regular, controlled ocular-motor movement. I ask a child to move their eyes in specific directions, follow objects visually, or closely observe how their eyes move during play. We may play games that involve specific eye movements at specific phases of therapy. If the therapy is working for them, I expect to see smoother, more coordinated, more effective eye movements. I also expect to see smoother and more coordinated movements, not just in the eyes but throughout the body, in various situations. If a child is incorporating vestibular awareness in their daily movements, games and interactions are safer, because he can anticipate others' movements better. He is more independent because he can imitate another person's actions to "do it myself."

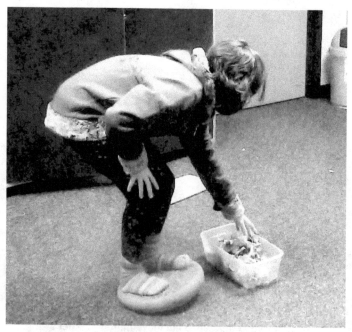

Fig. 1-4a: A child incorporating heightened vestibular awareness into movement.

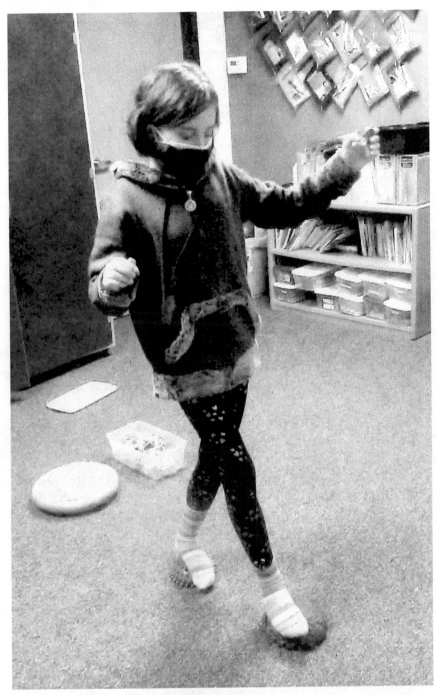

Fig. 1-4b: A child incorporating heightened vestibular awareness into movement.

Auditory Treatment

In her book *Eurythmics for Autism and Other Neurophysiologic Disorders*, Dorita Berger, a music therapist, strikes at the essence of the role of sound-based interventions. "So there are programs devised that enable the 'peg' [the **neurodiverse** person] to fit in (e.g.: ABA, TEACCH, Floortime, RDI, SCERTS)... The goal in music-based treatment is not to 'cure', but to reshape the 'peg'... to develop functional ways of managing behaviors" (p.78).

Auditory treatment is the therapeutic use of specific, electronically enhanced music and sounds. Music affects us all: we use it to soothe, such as quiet music to lull a baby to sleep; we use it to communicate emotion, such as a movie soundtrack that conveys fear in a scary scene; we use if to coordinate or stimulate movement, such as when we turn on our tunes to get us through an exercise session. It can socially bind us to others through shared musical experience. All of these natural elements of music, as well as others, can be used to help children normalize their motor coordination, communication, and emotional and biological regulation.

The auditory therapy system I chose to use in my clinic is called Therapeutic Listening©. It was developed by an OT, has a wide variety of album choices that address many different auditory-related issues, and is fairly economical. Ideally, I choose a specific album based on the child's needs and they listen to this album over the course of a week or two, twice a day, for 30 minute sessions. During each thirty-minute listening session, the child has many opportunities to practice the listening skill we are trying to evoke. The use of headphones is essential; having the sound physically proximal to them discourages them "tuning it out." The headphones I use are perforated, so the child can stay engaged in their surroundings and practice moving their attention to what draws it, both within the music and in their physical world. In essence, they are practicing "tuning in" and "filtering out."

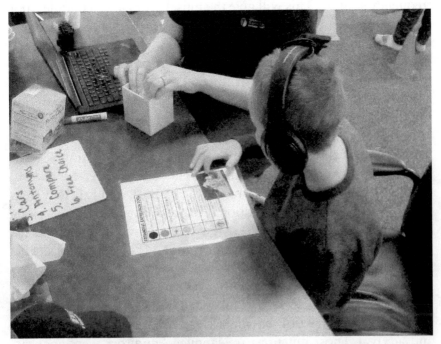

Fig. 1-5: A child "practices" listening during speech therapy.

Therapeutic Listening seems to increase the speed of their auditory processing. This can help with speech comprehension. In American English, there are an average of thirteen different sounds in speech per second. Understanding vocal pitch and emotional content as well as individual words means our brains are very busy when listening to someone speak. If a child has delayed auditory processing, their brains will be busy processing the *sounds* of speech, but might miss the meaning of what is being said.

Just as the child's response to vestibular input during assessment and treatment guides the therapeutic choices I make, my observations and parent information help me create an auditory therapy regimen unique to each child. I choose the music or sounds presented in the headphones based on the child's therapeutic needs, the inherent elements of the music or sounds, and what skill the sounds are meant to evoke. For example, a child (let's call him Dave) who is just beginning auditory therapy, has a medical history that includes chronic allergies and difficulty understanding speech sounds. Dave will likely need to begin with an album of simple music with a high contrast between high frequency and low frequency sounds. This will give the muscles of Dave's middle ear a chance to practice attuning to the frequencies presented. After one to two weeks, we should see an increased understanding of speech or an increase in attention when someone is speaking. It is then time to add complexity, such as instrumental music or stronger rhythms.

Let's continue with this same child. He has now begun to follow simple directions, but he still has trouble expressing himself and has tantrums instead of asking for what he wants. I might consider adding instrumental music to Dave's program. According to professor of Psychology Aniruddh Patel, instruments can be super-expressive, reaching registers that the human voice cannot, and this may help Dave's ear tune into the emotional expression created by various vocal pitch patterns. In the next few weeks, I would expect to see that Dave no longer has as many tantrums and can communicate his needs and emotions more clearly.

Auditory therapy is essentially using music and sounds to tap into what psychologist Steven Pinker calls the five non-musical brain functions, each function having a clear role in human adaptation and survival. Those functions are: language, auditory scene analysis, emotional processing and vocalization, habitat selection (wanting to stay in a safe place), and motor control. None of these functions is directly related to music, *per se*, but Pinker suggests that we derive pleasure from listening to music because it enhances the development of our ability to adapt and survive through our auditory sense.

The healthily skeptical reader may ask, "How do we know that *this specific* music is actually helping make the appropriate neural connections in a child's brain? How do we even know what neural connections are missing or wrong?" These are fair questions. Aside from the behavioral and functional improvements that I see in the clinic (which to me is the best yard-stick of this therapy's efficacy), there is no other way to concretely demonstrate neurological change. Study of the brain and human auditory processing has been limited to lesion studies, imaging technology and studying the results of epilepsy surgery. None of those methods of empirical data collection lend themselves to study in children. However, in studying adults, who we can put in imaging scanners, and animals, whose brains we can physically study, we do know that neural projections run both *to and from* the auditory cortex, the cochlea, the supportive musculature and neurological structures. It would stand to reason that, just like practicing the piano creates muscular and neurological changes in the hands, arms and brain, the structures of the ear and brain would also respond to repeated "listening" practice.

Author's Note

Throughout the book, I tell stories about children I have seen in the clinic to help me elucidate concepts, provide clinical examples, or demonstrate a chain of thought. Each of these children shone the light of knowledge for me. All of the stories are from actual cases, but the personal details and names have been changed. I am, and will always be, grateful to the children and families I've had the privilege to know over the years. I hope, if they read this book, that they might recognize their own stories and appreciate how their child helped other children by teaching me so well. I am so very lucky to have known each of them.

2 Yes, But How Do we *KNOW?*

"We must look at learning as the product of educational
self-organization."

—Sugata Mitra

I have been an occupational therapist (OT) for 20 years and worked
with children for over half that time. When I transferred from adults
to pediatrics, I had no idea what I was doing. I had briefly learned
about **sensory integration treatment** in OT school. I knew that it
was a specialty of OT practice and a framework for understanding
children's behavior and difficulties at a neurological level. Children
who need sensory integration treatment have trouble with daily
activities because they process bodily sensations abnormally. I
wanted to do my best for the children I would be treating, so I read
books and attended workshops about sensory problems in children.
Clinically, I experimented with suggestions for addressing sensory
problems from those books and workshops; such as sensory
exposure using water-based toys, bins full of rice or shaving foam
on mirrors.

To the parents with whom I worked, I parroted the same suggestions for increasing sleep or dealing with problems behaviors; warm
baths, consistent bedtime routines, using weighted vests or blankets.
I modeled techniques for increasing eye contact with my children
with autism; physical modeling and hand-over-hand guidance,
engaged play, and discreet trials (an attempt to elicit a desired
response in exchange for something the child likes). All those
methods worked for some children... a little bit. But no book or
workshop truly explained *why* children with autism, ADHD, learning difficulties, or sensory processing problems were different. No
source I encountered explained why I might choose one method
over another or what to do when nothing seemed to work.

Most importantly to me, nothing I tried in my first year of working with children provided the rapid results I wanted to see. I wanted results so evident that I would know *for certain* that what I was doing was helping children adapt to their world. Because if I wasn't helping a child make concrete, functional changes in their abilities, then I was wasting families' precious time.

Everything I tried felt as if I was putting out little fires, but not addressing the big blaze. A child would have a definitive deficit that affected their family, such as, "Timmy won't sit for more than three minutes, so we can never have a family meal together." I would offer suggestions specific to mealtimes for the family to try, given what I thought might be making it difficult for Timmy to sit still. I felt as if I was offering solutions to individual problems a child had, like so many "band-aids" to place over the outside, without understanding the problems each child was facing on the inside. I didn't really understand how to help children interact with their world more functionally, from within themselves.

A large part of my frustration was knowing that I had no more knowledge about how to help a child than their parents or teachers. Parents are the experts on their children. Why were they bringing their children to me? What could I possibly suggest or add that they had not researched on the internet, considered or tried on their own?

By way of example, a parent might ask, "Can you help my child learn to tie their shoes?" When a child ties their own shoes, they have a sense of accomplishment, are more independent, and free up precious moments of time from a harried parent. I desperately wanted a child to be able to tie their shoes. However, other than repeating the tying procedure *ad nauseum* (for both of myself and the child), I had no idea how to teach a child to tie their shoes, or more accurately, to *get a child to learn* to tie their shoes. What I needed to know was how to help a child to *teach themselves* how to tie their shoes. This is how all children learn new skills; they observe, possibly with an explanation from a more experienced person, then they are let loose on the field to build the skills from the ground up.

Children can't teach themselves to tie their shoes if they lack the requisite skills of attention, visual control, finger isolation, fine motor control, reach and grasp, ability to sequence, an understanding of perspective (to translate the viewing of how I tie *my* shoe to how theirs might look), and finally, the ability to critique their own work to evaluate success and learn from failure. Say what? How am I going to help a child with ALL THAT!? That was an extremely tall order when I only had an hour or two each week with any given child. Even as a professional with a good understanding of human development, I still felt lost and ineffective. Parents were bringing their children to me for help, and I felt like I couldn't offer them anything unique, effective and of true value in their lives.

I was reaching the point of feeling that transferring to pediatrics was a mistake, when I took a continuing education course on auditory therapy. It was my introduction into how important the **auditory** (listening *and* looking) **system** and **vestibular** (balance and movement) **system** are in everything we do as functional human beings. During the course, I was jotting notes furiously as light bulbs were popping in my head, connecting the theory on which auditory therapy is based to the individual children I was trying to help. These theories explained so many of the behaviors I didn't understand and felt unable to help my children with.

However, understanding what might be wrong in a child's wiring and being able to help them straighten out the wires are two very different things. Was this therapy effective in treating what might be the actual problem for a given child? By the time I returned to the clinic, I was dubious that one particular intervention could accomplish everything that auditory therapy seemed to promise; better motor control, fewer disruptive behaviors, greater comprehension and flexibility of ideas—the list went on and on. I'm a natural skeptic, and until I've reproduced results myself, I never quite believe what's promised.

Clinton Anderson, a noted horse trainer, says, "Your frustration begins when your knowledge ends." After the auditory-therapy course, I continued to work with a wonderful boy with autism who was whip-smart, funny, and loving. My frustration with treating him was definitely growing, because I had reached the end of my knowledge regarding how to help him communicate, tolerate noises around him and behave more functionally. He was a perfect test subject with whom to try something new and hopefully expand my knowledge.

At only five-years-old, Brandon had been in occupational, speech and physical therapy for years. When he was diagnosed with autism, his mother Susan immediately sought out all the therapies recommended by Brandon's doctor. She followed all of the recommendations of those therapists, as much as a mother with another son and a household to think about possibly could. While Brandon did not speak, he had found ways to communicate his intelligence, sense of humor, and needs by laughing, sometimes drawing intricate pictures of what he wanted. He was an extraordinary boy with a devoted, but completely no-nonsense mother. Despite years of treatment, he remained unable to speak and he was often frustrated by his inability to communicate. He had strong emotional tantrum reactions, particularly to sounds and crowds, limiting his ability to participate in school and at home. In the six months I had been working with him, we had made almost no progress.

I knew I had reached the limit of my abilities to help Brandon. We lived in an area with very limited options for therapy and there was no one with more experience to refer Brandon's mother. Ethically, I couldn't continue to see Brandon when progress seemed unlikely, but I had no alternative to offer. It felt like a dead-end. It was with anxiety and sadness that I confessed to his mother that I wouldn't be able to continue seeing Brandon because we had reached what the therapy world refers to as a "plateau." I knew that, at least for the immediate future, this version of Brandon was as functional as I knew how to help him be. The best hope I could offer was the possibility that, after some time to mature, he might be ready to learn additional skills or new routines.

However, at the workshop I'd just attended I had purchased some of the requisite equipment to administer auditory therapy. While I knew Brandon tended to be overly sensitive to sounds, I had no idea what this therapy might do for him. "Susan," I said, "I have these headphones and a couple of CDs that I just learned how to use. While I won't see Brandon clinically anymore, I could prescribe a listening program. If you're willing to learn to help him listen through the headphones at home on a schedule, you and I can touch base when he's here for other therapy appointments, you can tell me how it's going. If you want to continue with it, we can adapt the program as he needs it." Being game to try anything that might help her son, she agreed and took the equipment home that day.

The following week, she and Brandon arrived for a speech therapy appointment. Susan took Brandon's hand and almost ran up to me in the hallway. "Robin! Robin! You have GOT to hear this!" Then she leaned down toward her son and said, "The sheep in the field say..." With the air of a child who had put this particular skill on display too many times for his liking, he rolled his eyes skyward and said, "Baa." I lit up! At five-years-old, Brandon's first word was "baa"! I hugged Susan and we laughed with glee. She asked for another CD and we proceeded to take Brandon through a few more albums.

What was this miracle? Would it work for other children? Was Brandon just primed to speak anyway, or was it the auditory therapy that made the difference? In my naiveté, I did not resume therapy with Brandon, but now I know better. Had I added additional types of auditory therapy and regimented therapy for his vestibular system, I believe his results would have been even more robust. As it was, Brandon did learn to speak, but at the time I last saw him (when he was around eight years of age) his verbal communication remained limited to expression of what he needed and didn't include emotional expression or an ability to communicate about his internal landscape.

Over the next several months, I added more "miracle" stories to my experience with auditory therapy; more first words, a nine-year-old who could calmly tolerate a trip to the store with her mother for the first time after a listening session, a little boy who independently says "I love you" to his mother, and for the first time she realizes that he's not parroting her words back to her, but expressing real emotion.

This was amazing! As I learned more, I added another component to my therapy; regimented, controlled vestibular therapy. The vestibular system, like the auditory system, is housed in the inner ear. It helps us understand our position in space and whether or not we are moving. This additional treatment seemed to create a new dimension of progress for many children; their eyes moved around their environment more easily, they gained confidence and ease in movement; some began to be able to dress themselves or have fewer tantrums.

Concurrent with my elation at making a meaningful difference in families' lives was an overwhelming frustration with other free-standing, and seemingly less effective, types of therapy, and with professionals who didn't incorporate knowledge of the auditory and vestibular systems into their therapy practice. However, it occurred to me that, if I hadn't already known about these therapies going into my post-professional master's program, I wouldn't have known about them as a result of the program, either. They were never mentioned; so other professionals might not know how or why to incorporate them into their therapy.

If professionals had to be introduced to this information seemingly by chance, how could parents possibly be expected to stumble upon it when they are overwhelmed by a child's behaviors or new diagnosis? Even with the advent of the internet, I've had parents tell me this was nowhere to be found in the thousands of articles and blog posts they had scoured looking for help and answers.

I found this lack of access to information for people who were desperate for it both frustrating and heart-breaking. It became a mission for me to help families and other professionals understand how these treatments could help their child. As I explained how the auditory and vestibular systems impact development the within the womb and onward, I found parents asking insightful questions and wanting to hear more. I could see the parents expanding these ideas from their child, to themselves and their spouses. Applying these developmental ideas to themselves helped parents better empathize with their child. Why do we choose certain activities or have certain preferences that are different from others? Why are some people night owls and some morning people? Why do some people become computer programmers and others become rock stars? Our need for, and tolerance of, sound and movement is the basis for so many life choices. It is comforting to know why *we* are the way *we* are, and even more comforting to realize why your child may be different.

The Four Arenas of Time and Space

Before we explore how we navigate the space around us and why we make certain choices, we need to share a common way to think about our environment. Our function in the world around us is not just impacted by the room we are in, but it's also our internal sensations, our thoughts and memories, our unique interpretation of sensation, and how all of those things interact with each other. At any given moment in time, our mental energy is spent attending to our situation in one of four distinct categories of time and space. Our ability to function throughout our day is dependent on our ability to move in and out of these four areas of time and space as required for each activity in which we need to participate. The four arenas are:

Body time and space: You are in body space and time when you are: stretching after sitting for a long while, registering the sensation of having to use the restroom, or exercising. There are times when our visit into body space is brief, such as when we touch something soft and fuzzy. A functional person should be able to leave body space quite easily to attend to the world around them, but there are times when the body's need for attention intrudes on our ability to do other things, such as when we are hungry and we cannot ignore the feeling of hunger to concentrate in a meeting.

Near time and space: You are operating in near time and space when you are: typing on the computer, preparing a meal, or completing your morning care routine at the sink. The tasks of near time and space tend to be finite. You have everything you need for the task, there is usually a logical sequence of events, and you end your participation because the task is completed. We often hang out longer in near time and space when we are participating in craft-type hobbies and we lose track of time. There are times when our attention is taken away from near space and time and we cannot complete an activity easily or well, such as when we become lost in thought in the shower and realize that we have not finished rinsing the shampoo out of our hair before turning off the water (not that that has ever happened to me).

Far time and space: This arena of time and space could be: attending to the instructor during a class, driving a car, or playing a ball sport. While watching a truly engrossing movie, we can stay very absorbed in far time and space. When we become injured while playing a sport, we are brought very quickly and abruptly *out* of far time and space, and into body space to attend to our needs.

Mental time and space: As adults, we spend quite a bit of time in mental time and space; planning our days, remembering past events, and creating solutions to problems. This can be a productive arena, allowing us to be imaginative and creative, but it can also create difficulties; keeping us trapped in our minds, repeating unproductive thoughts and obsessions. This is why yoga and exercise are good for stress reduction and decreasing anxiety; we return to body space and time in the moment, and escape anxiety-provoking obsessive thoughts in mental space and time.

Consider your child's behavior throughout a typical day and see if you can figure out in which sphere of space and time they prefer to be. Do they have trouble moving from one category of space and time to another? It could be likely that their predominant place in space and time might not be a good enough fit for the activity we would like them to do, or the activity they need to participate in for functional development.

If a child is predominately spending time in near space, which can happen for a variety of reasons we will explore in this book, they will miss opportunities for social interaction, physical play, or mental space activities such as imagining, all of which are crucial for development. If a child is predominately in mental space, he may not be able to hear new sounds in the environment—he misses looking at people's faces to make emotional connections, and may fail to associate the proper visual image with auditory information. Typically, these sound-vision connections are to words and feelings; the primary way in which we all learn language. Opportunities for visual attention, which close this "loop of learning", are becoming less frequent for children due to the proliferation of screens in our culture. Television and videogame screens give constant incentives for a child to keep their eyes locked in one place, losing opportunities to move their eyes, practice orienting to new information, and communicate fully with others.

The Orienting Response and Sensory Mismatch

The physiological function that allows us to move between spheres of time and space is the **orienting response**. When some sensation or thought catches our attention, our brain automatically assesses that new information, asking, "What is this new thought or feeling?" If our orienting response is functional, our brain attends to the stimulus, further asking "Am I familiar with it? Is it safe? Is it relevant to what I am doing?" The brain does this by making a sensory match or mismatch. If there is a sensory match, the brain then decides whether to create a motor response to address the stimulus.

A Simple Task

To better understand the concept of changing arenas of time and space, at will and as necessary, I thought I would break-down a task we all do several times a day in terms of the time and space awareness arenas; going to the bathroom. Let's look at just a few aspects of this task that neurotypical people master by about age 3. To use the restroom, one must:

1. Recognize the sensation of needing to "go," involving body awareness (*feeling* the sensation) and mental space (*recognizing* it as the sensation that means bladder fullness).

2. Adjust the course of your day to make time to go, involving awareness of how long the task will take and whether there are any more pressing tasks that need attention first (a mental time and space activity).

3. Locate the restroom and fixtures, involving the mental space of navigation, the far space of visual location, and the near space of finding an unoccupied stall.

4. Have the physical control to interact with the environment (wiping, flushing, etc.), involving body space and near space awareness.

This list is just a few of the myriad tasks involved in a "simple" activity, and yet each involves adjusting one's focus and attention by allowing it to flow from one arena of time and space to another, in an overlapping dance of sensation and thought; which is remarkable, as most of us complete the entire task without much conscious thought.

If it is a familiar noise, like the clack of computer keys from our spouse working in their home office, we will likely not have a motor response, not even looking up in answer to the noise because we know what it is. If there is a sensory match to a familiar noise that *does* require a motor response, such as when we hear our child crying, then our conscious mind engages to develop an appropriate motor plan.

What if there's a sensory mismatch? Then, our attention is drawn more deeply into the stimulus. For example, if you have heard your husband typing away in his office, and your brain has filtered out that sound (a process called **habituation**, which we will explore), but then you hear a crash and a curse, your brain makes a sensory mismatch and this creates an alert in your brain and body. You were not expecting such an unusual noise from the activity of someone typing, so your attention is held on the stimulus to investigate it. You might call out, "Is everything alright?" or get up from the couch to see for yourself.

Our Internal Gyroscope

Remember back in school when you were learning about fractions? Remember what the lowest common denominator was? It was the number of "pieces" a fraction should be divided into so that all the "pieces" would be the same size. It was the magic number that made all the different fractions part of the same language. It was what they all had in common.

Learning is a bit like that. We take in little pieces of knowledge; little packets of information. We tend to think of learning as a linear, continuous process. Like sitting in a classroom or learning to drive. Someone "gives" us the lesson or we learn the basic skills, and we continue to build more knowledge and skills on top of what someone else taught us. That's a very well-developed, adult conception of learning. For babies and children, learning takes place in much smaller doses, because their skills are just starting to be developed. But the common denominator for all these ways of learning, the thing all learning experiences have in common, is the orienting response.

The orienting response is the first moment that must happen in any learning experience, or else nothing will be learned. Even if you are learning about things you don't like: that astrophysics bores

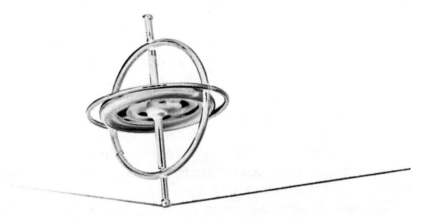

Fig. 2-1: A gyroscope maintains its center of balance no matter how the earth shifts beneath it

you, that the harpsichord makes a sound you can't stand, or that stubbing your toe hurts in a certain way. The orienting response happens in a fraction of a second, but it *must* happen to gain our attention to a stimulus so that learning can occur. The orienting response occurs for every one of us thousands of times each day. We experience the orienting response every time something catches our attention. It might be a visual stimulus, such as seeing something move across our visual field. Because our visual field is only about 150 degrees of our 360-degree environment, the stimulus that triggers our attention is more likely to be a sound or a feeling. If your nervous system is functioning properly, it filters out irrelevant sensations. Consequently, the sensation that piques the orienting response will be a relevant sensation in that situation, alerting you that something new has occurred in your environment.

For example, you are watching TV while your kids play nearby. Your brain has already been filtering out the sound of their play so you can focus on the television program, when the doorbell rings. That is a new noise within the space, and before you even begin to move off the couch to answer the door, your brain and body experience the orienting response. First, your brain registers the stimulus as new, and therefore worthy of your attention. Then there is a momentary stilling of the body and breath, and a resulting brief drop in heart rate. In a functional adult, this is often so brief that it is really unnoticeable. But when a young child is confronted by a novel stimulus, it's a fairly obvious moment: they stop. Moving back to the doorbell example, your brain analyzes where the sound is coming from and your core muscles activate to provide a stable base around which to pivot your head and body toward the source of this noise. You may not even look toward the door because your previous experience has taught you that there will be no new visual information there until the door is opened. All of this takes place in the space of a fraction of a second. The orienting response is what allows us to answer the question, "What is this new thing?" and to prepare an appropriate motor response; answer the door or turn off the lights and pretend not to be home.

To understand what might be wrong for a person whose orienting response is dysfunctional, we must first understand what allows a functional orienting response to take place. For the orienting response to happen correctly for us, we must already have knowledge of our situation in two distinct ways. One, we must be aware of the space that surrounds us: how large or small it is, and who or what is in it. Two, we must be aware of our position in that space: how much space is behind us, what our physical posture is, and that our physical position in space is unique to us and no one else can occupy this specific space in this specific moment in time.

How do we know all of these things about the space around us and our position in it? We each have an internal gyroscope. A gyroscope is a structure of rotating disks which, when in motion, provide stability in relation to earth's gravity, no matter how the mount on which it rests moves. It provides a point of reference to allow for changes in direction with both stability and mobility, independent of external influences.

Our internal gyroscope gives us our orientation, using sensations picked up by the vestibular system and the auditory system. Our vestibular system gives us our orientation in gravity-bound space, and our auditory system gives us an initial understanding of the relevant information within that space. Put another way: *One's vestibular sense is the first influence on the development of understanding of position in space. One's auditory sense is the first influence on the development of understanding of the space and time in which one is.* Two structures of the inner ear, the **vestibulum** and the **cochlea**, are the sensory organs for these systems. They function as every person's first global positioning system; telling them where they are, where they are going, and what's nearby. The other senses like touch and sight must correspond what the inner ear already knows, or dysfunction results. And just like when the GPS in your car or your phone goes on the fritz while you're in unfamiliar territory; in the absence of guidance you can become disoriented, anxious and frustrated.

The orienting response is essentially constructed on these two systems; the vestibular and auditory systems. The auditory sense is fully formed in the womb, and infants in the womb hear their mother's voice. Babies orient to mother's voice very shortly after birth; because of the sensory-match to previous knowledge created while *in utero*. Also in the womb, a fetus's fully-developed vestibular sense begins to tell it when it is moving and when it is stationary. Because of these experiences, after birth a baby will know he is stationary, lying on his blanket without moving, as he hears his mother's voice. He begins to develop the motor control to stabilize his head and neck, to direct his eyes toward her voice because he first knows he is stable in space, thanks to the vestibular information he learned before he was born. Learning to control his eyes, learning where sensations in his body arise from, and how to control his muscles will occur based on already acquired knowledge from his functional vestibular and auditory systems.

For typically-developing persons, these two systems create the foundational structure on which all subsequent learning about their environment is based.

The vestibular systems help all of us:

- create a "ground-zero" for our construct of the space around us and our position in it, giving us the "You Are Here" cue in a given space.

- inform our emotional brain centers to tell us we are physically safe.

- direct our attention to stimuli around us, and filter out what is irrelevant.

- sequence events and objects (e.g. counting, patterns, etc.)

- coordinate our eyes and bodies for effective interaction with our physical environment.

The auditory system plays a key role in:

- awareness of the size and shape of the space around us.

- orienting to new stimuli.

- alerting us to dangers; it is our "early warning" system.

- our internal concept of time, sequence and rhythm.

If a child's auditory and vestibular senses are functioning properly, their orienting response will help them develop a consistent database of experiences to make sensory matches or mismatches—to recognize a sensation as something already known and safe, or something unknown and then potentially dangerous or interesting. Remember, the orienting response helps answer the questions "What is this new thing? Is this new thing safe?" To do that, we must have a set of data about the world to draw from and make comparisons to.

What Auditory and Vestibular Treatment is Called

As you'll read in this book, there are many different programs of vestibular and auditory treatment. I treat both the vestibular and auditory systems of all the children I see using methods that *I* like, but other therapists may use different methods to address the same systems. The important thing is that these systems *are* addressed in therapy, first and foremost. Saying "auditory and vestibular systems" or "auditory and vestibular treatment" can be cumbersome, so this type of therapy can be referred to differently in different arenas. It's a good idea to ask your child's therapist how he is addressing these systems, if he has a standardized approach or treatment program, and what the name of that program is, so that you can do some research on your own.

However, expected patterns of auditory and vestibular development might be derailed by many factors: maternal physical stress or poor nutrition during gestation, premature or breech birth, lack of emotionally-supportive contact or extended NICU stays after birth, or any number of other things. In my experience, occasionally there is no red-herring event or circumstance. In these cases, difficulties in a child's orienting response and sensation database can still be treated effectively. Through specific therapy targeting these systems, sensations can become consistent within their sensory world, giving a child a consistent set of data for inferences and deductions.

As parents come to understand why they attend to stimuli, and therefore learn, they understand their children better. It is especially difficult to understand the motivations and choices of people with autism, attention-deficit hyperactivity disorder (ADHD) and sensory processing disorder (SPD) because their bodies and brains operate so differently from **neurotypical** people. Our "guides" into the world of autism, people with these differences themselves, can only explain how certain behaviors make them feel or help them navigate their world. They cannot articulate, from a developmental perspective, *why* they choose to perform those particular behaviors. The gift of people with autism like Temple Grandin and Naoki Hisgashida has been their ability to explain to neurotypical people how certain behaviors make them feel. Temple Grandin has enlightened her readers about how an autistic person's brain might perceive the world differently. But, as insightful as her work has been, she is unable to explain *why* her brain's perception is different and how her brain became so uniquely wired.

Starting at the Beginning

Many children diagnosed with autism, ADHD, or developmental delays enter the occupational, physical or speech therapist's office for the first time at the age of three or older. Perhaps the child had a history of being a "challenging" infant or toddler, but her parents found ways to cope. Perhaps the child was independent and capable at home with mom, but when he entered school, educators became concerned regarding his ability to absorb new information or adapt to a new way of doing tasks. Sometimes, a child may seem to be developing normally, only to lose skills later as autism takes hold.

Regardless, because children may come into the therapist's office walking and possibly talking, it is easy to assume that the developmental mechanisms that helped them achieve walking and talking did a "good enough" job, and that therapists can't, or don't need to, address these mechanisms. We assume that adjusting a child's current function is all that is necessary or possible. For example, if a child appears to have decreased balance in standing, a therapist is likely to help the child develop better balance through tasks that involve standing and balancing. But a therapist addressing the development of balance will work on helping a child *sense* movement and equilibrium without asking for a motor response. This is the developmental sequence for all of us, as we were moved through space by our parents before and after birth.

In a traditional approach to therapy, parents may be taught to help their child by using practice techniques and drills, compensation techniques, or special equipment. In illustration, the likely conclusion regarding a child who is four-years-old but cannot scoop pudding with a spoon, is that she has fine-motor deficits. Traditionally-accepted therapy would work on her fine-motor skills, such as eating practice and table-top games. The child who constantly knocks things over while playing has **proprioceptive** (body and muscle awareness) difficulties, so coordination activities may be prescribed. The child who cannot climb the stairs without pulling up on a banister has weak leg muscles, so strengthening exercises are taught to him and his family.

I propose that, quite often therapists are not necessarily working on the *wrong* things, but starting in the wrong place. Practicing the skill the child *cannot* do would seem to be the logical treatment in helping the child master it. But first we must address the underlying problem that originally created difficulty in mastering those skills. Perhaps the child who cannot climb the stairs may have perfectly strong legs, but cannot sense when his center of gravity is over his stepping leg, or his brain cannot estimate how hard to push. Both of these skills are built on a functional, accurate vestibular system. Working on this skill through practice without addressing his vestibular dysfunction will not help him easily adjust when the stairs are new and different; with carpet or different height steps.

Treating the vestibular and auditory needs of the child at the outset of intervention addresses the root of why certain skills are overly-difficult for the child. This treatment helps to "straighten out" neural pathways that began to form from before birth. Because children's brains are in a constant state of neural growth and elimination, neurons that were pruned when they should have been strengthened or strengthened when they should have been pruned can create dysfunctional patterns of behavior. Although the child may be five years old, walking and talking, the child's current struggles likely began much earlier in their lives. They may have developed the skills that they have by compensating in a variety of ways, but the wires are still crossed.

A New Conception of Learning

I believe most people conceive of learning something along the lines of the illustration in Fig. 2-2. This hierarchy places the traditional "five senses" (minus "smell"), augmented by vestibular and proprioceptive (joint movement awareness) senses, at the base, and assumes that learning is built on the foundation of these senses. At the very bottom of the pyramid is the base that assumes children feel things with their bodies first, then connect to the outside world.

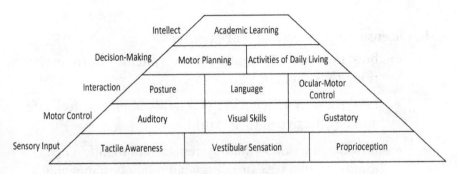

Fig. 2-2: Old "Pyramid of Learning."

In this model, the vestibular system *does* play a significant role in the foundation for learning preparation. However, the vestibular and auditory systems are fully functional in the womb and *at* birth, and the vision, tactile and proprioceptive systems develop predominately *after* birth. In my estimation, a child feels the outside world first through movement and sound, as it influences his or her body. The human body is unlikely to begin to incorporate learning from a system that is not fully developed yet, and is instead going to use the fully-developed auditory and vestibular systems to make sense of its surroundings. It stands to reason that any complication or dysfunction in these two systems would create a cascade of difficulties in higher functions of the body and brain. Therefore, a more accurate conception of how we learn may look more like Fig. 2-3:

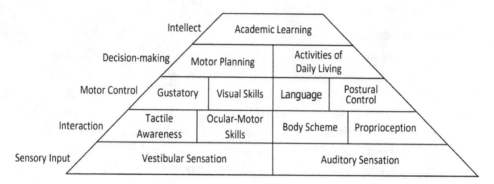

Fig. 2-3: New "Pyramid of Learning."

In the ensuing chapters, we will explore:

- how the vestibular and auditory systems inform everything that children learn.

- how these systems affect children's ability to feel safe and be effective in their world.

- how dysfunction in these systems might manifest behaviorally, so that we can assess what might be happening in a child's brain and help them to re-wire their brain to respond more functionally.

As we discuss the anatomy and physiology of the auditory and vestibular system throughout this book, you may become a bit overwhelmed if your background does not include classes on anatomy. It is less important for you to understand the physiology of these systems, than to recognize what might be wrong based on a child's behavior and responses.

How a child experiences sound and movement plays a paramount role in early development. If we understand the preeminence of these systems, it becomes easier to understand how the chain of events that *should* occur can be altered when auditory and vestibular development are negatively impacted. Because we cannot flip open children's little heads to observe exactly where their neural impulses are going, we have to rely on their behaviors to help us piece together the puzzle of what they are experiencing internally. Throughout this book, I will try to give concrete examples, both clinical cases I've encountered and examples of how your own systems function and malfunction (and that happens to all of us). Hopefully, these examples will make the concepts understandable and pliable for you. And with that understanding, you can begin to understand and help your child.

3   The Art of Noise

While children come to my clinic with a range of difficulties, one of the most stressful and frustrating for parents is when a child over the age of two isn't developing verbal communication skills. Development of verbal communication depends on an understanding of the emotional content in speech, as delivered through vocal harmonics and pitch, aspects of time in speech, such as cadence and pauses, and sound localization of speech, so that the child can look at a person's face and mouth. With a basic understanding of auditory development and neurology from this chapter, we can begin to delve into the specifics of how these skills develop in the next couple of chapters.

But before we do, I'd like to answer the question that I was stumped by before I began to explore these concepts clinically. I skeptically wondered, "Well, it's interesting, all this auditory function and how it supports cognitive and communication development. But, can a therapist actually help a child's auditory sense develop further and help the child function better?" Enter auditory therapy.

Most auditory therapy programs are designed based on the same principles, initially developed by Dr. Alfred Tomatis, a French otolaryngologist in the 1950s. He was simultaneously treating opera singers who had lost certain vocal ranges in their singing, and factory workers who had lost the hearing of specific pitches due to their work. From this work, he developed his process of auditory therapy; using recorded sounds and a person's own vocal feedback. He developed the idea that listening could be rehabilitated through exposure to specific, emphasized sounds.

Since that time, modern recording and sound-engineering methods have allowed developers and practitioners of auditory therapy to experiment with electronically-modified sound. In most every type of auditory therapy, music (instrumental, vocal or synthesized) and/or natural sounds are recorded, and sometimes electronically altered, for playback through high-quality headphones. A knowledgeable practitioner can assign the sounds that might be necessary to help the ear develop or recover specific function. This is accomplished both through music's role for all of us (rhythm, social cohesion, emotional expression), as well as repeated exposure to orienting sounds in a close environment (the nearness of the headphones making it easier to attend to sound). Because near-sound is easier to orient and attend to, a single session of auditory therapy presents multiple opportunities for a child to practice processing sound for recognition and sequencing in a slower-paced process.

In the clinic, this might look like a child involved in a play activity while wearing a set of headphones playing the prescribed auditory therapy. A child might also be prescribed a set time and pattern of participation in auditory therapy outside the clinic as well. Those details depend on the child's needs and the therapist's treatment approach. However, in most cases, auditory therapy is an adjunct treatment—a component of therapy that supports or happens simultaneously during other, more engaging activities.

Almost anyone can use auditory therapy to help children, be that person an occupational therapist, speech therapist, teacher, or parent—anyone can take classes and become certified in one of several different types of sound therapy. A competent auditory therapist must consider many aspects of sound and their effect on the brain using a complex series of clinical decisions. Some programs are designed in sequence, taking the artistry out of the application, but eventually allowing a child to hear the sounds that are rehabilitative for them specificially.

The Function of Listening

Our sense of hearing, combined with our database of previous experiences, lets us analyze our situation and make decisions with speed and accuracy. Consider this example: You are doing dishes at the sink, and your children are playing somewhere in the house. Suddenly you hear a loud noise. Instantly, you analyze that noise without conscious thought. Was it a thud, like piece of furniture falling over, or a crash, like a lamp being broken? Where in the house did it come from? It is followed by a child's cry? Have you heard it before, when the children were jumping off the bed? All these questions, asked by your brain subconsciously, help you decide within a second if you need to go check out the noise and see if anyone is hurt, or maybe just yell at your kids to stop horsing around in the house. Can you imagine what it would be like to have to investigate every noise you heard because your brain *did not* go through this process? The interruptions to life's daily activities would be compounded by the fact that we can't close our ears, as we can our eyes. Can you imagine how hard it would be to rest and relax if every noise was raised to a conscious level to be analyzed as "safe" or "unsafe"?

Our sense of hearing operates 24 hours of each day, even when we are asleep. Our lower, more primitive brain centers filter information coming into our ears and decide whether that information is important enough to raise to the level of consciousness. This is why we can sleep soundly when a train passes every night at midnight, but if our new baby snuffles for a moment, our eyes bolt open. Our brains are listening and sifting through many pieces of auditory information every second of the day, deciding what is important and deserves our attention and what is not. Because the auditory system often makes these decisions without our conscious involvement, its effect on our attention and alertness is often beyond our conscious control. Paying attention is something that even adults often have difficulty doing by conscious choice. It's virtually impossible for a child to attend to something when their brain has not developed to be able to recognize the relevant from the irrelevant.

We each have different threshold levels of attention to, and tolerance of, sounds. Because our responses to sound can be so different from one another, I believe they play a role in some of the decisions we make across the life span; whether we are introverts or extroverts, whether we become musicians or librarians, whether we want a large family or a small one. Listening is not passive. It is a process involving both intake and active modulation of responses that affects our response to the environment, the decisions we make, and why some talents or skills come more easily to some people, while they remain a struggle for others.

Two different people, both with 100% normal and functional hearing, might react very differently to the same to sound within their environment. I used to work with a person whose hearing was completely within normal levels of acuity, but his brain filtered out too many salient sounds while he was concentrating and would not alert him to changes around him. If I entered the office and said "Good Morning" he would practically jump out of his skin in surprise because he was startled. His brain didn't attend to the sound of me opening the door or to my footfalls, so I was much closer to him than he was aware of when his attention was finally caught by the sound of my voice; as if I had snuck up on him, but I was not making "sneaky" levels of sound. He is computer programmer, and a dedicated introvert. He can concentrate for long periods of time, oblivious to his environment. It's not a huge leap to guess that his difficulty sensing and responding calmly to his environment might have influenced his choice of activities he enjoys, and thus his career.

Personally, I have the opposite problem. All sounds seem to come in at the same volume for me. It is very difficult for me to tune out to the sounds of other people moving around, or dogs barking outside, or air conditioners cycling while I work. Over the years I have learned to employ ear plugs or soft background music when I need to concentrate. I've learned to avoid loud bars or restaurants when I want to have a conversation, and I never have the TV on unless watching it is the activity of the moment. As a child, I didn't have such self-awareness or ability to modify my environment, so it was very difficult for me to hear a teacher speaking over the normal classroom sounds of pencils scratching and chairs scooting. I would

---

Sound and Sleep

Children who are hypersensitive to sound while they are awake will most likely have trouble filtering out unimportant sounds while they are asleep as well. Thus, sounds like the air conditioner cycling on during the night awaken the child, even though their brain should have habituated to that noise as familiar and safe; it's just too darned loud. Children can benefit from having a source of ambient noise in the room with them to mask other noises that may be waking them. A fan, white-noise machine or soft music recording is preferable; not a TV or radio, as the noise from those sound sources can be varied and therefore alerting.

often find my attention wandering out the window as filtering the teacher's voice through the ambient sound became too taxing quite early in a lesson. In his book *When Listening Comes Alive*, Paul Madaule called this "the paradox of poor listening", that it really means one hears too much.

The Physiology of Listening

Before we explore what the ear does for us, let's first take a look at what the ear is, and how it works. There is some terminology to become familiar with as we go, but we'll start with a picture of the ear:

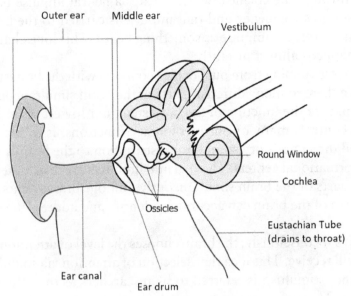

Fig. 3-1: Anatomy of the ear.

From left to right, the outer area, called the **pinna**, is the part of the ear we refer to from the outside, and it captures sound waves to be better directed into the ear canal. These sound waves "beat" the ear drum, and that vibration is transmitted through three tiny, feather-light bones called ossicles to the oval window of the inner ear (at the far-right end of the chain of bones).

The ossicles are housed in what is referred to as the middle ear. It has a tube called the eustachian tube that drains fluid from the middle ear into the throat. This is the biological mechanism that allows us to reset our ear drums to the appropriate tension as the atmosphere changes. We "pop" our ears by opening our eustachian tubes and equalizing the pressure on both sides of the ear drum as the atmospheric pressure changes (due to weather or altitude changes). The middle ear may become clogged when you are sick and mucous thickens. An increase in pressure in the middle ear due to an ear infection is what a doctor sees when they look into your ear and sees the eardrum reddened and convex, instead of its normal slightly concave.

Vibration leaves the ossicles and gets transmitted to the oval window at the end of the chain of bones. This oval window vibrates at the frequency of sound hitting the ear drum, and the vibration is carried through the cochlea, which creates a neural impulse based on the sound's frequency and that impulse is carried to the brain, which interprets the impulse as something heard. This long chain of events happens almost instantly.

The nerve running from our cochlea connects with the brainstem, and from there to many different parts of the brain simultaneously. In fact, part of the function of the brainstem, our lowest brain center that controls many of our involuntary functions, is to receive, filter and direct auditory stimuli for distribution to the brain's various informational centers. These neural impulses are distributed to various parts of the brain simultaneously, but our brains "choose" which area of the brain can accurately identify and address the new stimuli.

Often subconsciously, the brain chooses the level of attention the sound will receive. This idea that selection of attention via sound (or some other stimulus), is referred to by researchers as the "Reverse Hierarchy Theory" of perception (in this case, perception of sound). It purports that the same sound is repeatedly represented at various places in our brains, part of our **sound database** that we will explore throughout this book, and our brain subconsciously selects the level of representation that is relevant to the task at hand.

For example, the sound of footsteps in a busy office is a sound easily recognized. If you work in an open environment in which people are walking by all day, your brain filters this information out at a very low level of consciousness. It is not relevant to the task at hand—you completing your work. However, if you were working late into the evening and the office was very quiet, this same sound would be more alerting. This is because your brain has another, similar neural pattern representing "footsteps" at a higher level of consciousness. Hearing this noise late at night might mean the more relevant task is not to complete your work, but to interact with an approaching person. The representation within your brain of "approaching footsteps" becomes processed at higher brain levels because you need to be more alert to what the footsteps mean for you in that moment. This is the "hierarchy" to which the title of the theory refers; the information travels to any place in the brain that the sound might be relevant, but then lets the lowest level of the neurological totem pole take care of the response, depending on the situation.

These diffuse neural connections throughout the brain make the auditory sense a chief regulator of attention, helping the brain decide what information within our 360-degree surround to filter out and what information to attend. The auditory sense directs a dance between ignoring irrelevant information (a process called *habituation*) and *attention* to relevant information, thus creating the opportunity for learning.

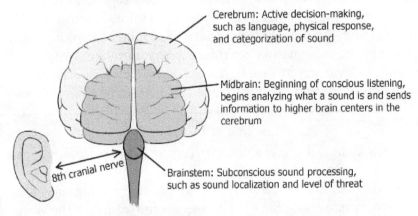

Cerebrum: Active decision-making, such as language, physical response, and categorization of sound

Midbrain: Beginning of conscious listening, begins analyzing what a sound is and sends information to higher brain centers in the cerebrum

8th cranial nerve

Brainstem: Subconscious sound processing, such as sound localization and level of threat

Fig. 1-2: Sound processing areas of the brain.

Listening Pathways in the Brain

Before sound can reach the brain as a neural impulse, it must first be processed by the ear from physical sound waves. You might remember from your high-school physics class that all sound is composed of the compression and expansion of particles in the air. This is why there is no sound in outer space; there's no atmosphere to compress or expand. The frequency of the air waves—how many peaks of each wave hit the ear drum per second—determines the

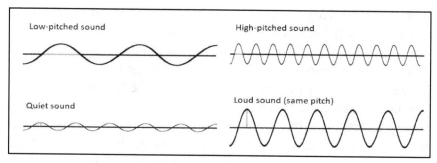

Fig. 3-3: Sound waves.

pitch of the tone the ear hears (see Fig 3-3). Higher frequencies have higher pitches and lower frequencies have lower pitches.

After a sound changes to a neural impulse in the ear, it travels along the 8th cranial (vestibulocochlear) nerve to the brainstem, which begins to filter the sound-information based on the timing, frequency match between ears and intensity, allowing the brain to develop an initial guess about where the sound is coming from. At the brainstem level the information is being processed by our unconscious mind, giving us a helping us to know *where* a sound is coming from, but not necessarily *what* the sound is. Evolutionarily-speaking, the information regarding *where* in our environment a potential threat might be—how far and in which direction—was more important to our survival, and the intervention of our slower

Looking at Listening

When a sound of a given pitch arrives at the ear drum, the ear drum vibrates to that frequency. Those vibrations are carried through three interconnected bones to another membrane called the oval window (see Fig 4). This membrane transmits the vibrations into the cochlea, which contains a long bed of tiny, hair-like cells that is coiled into a snail shape. Each section of that bed of cells responds to a different frequency within our range of hearing. When specific cells in this bed are activated by a specific frequency, they change that vibration into a neural impulse that is carried into the brain via the vestibulocochlear nerve. There's a wonderful video by Brandon Pletsch that you can find on YouTube that illustrates this process beautifully.

"thinking" brain to identify it specifically, meant the difference between life and death.

The neural impulses then move to the midbrain, where the reception of sound can lead to the orienting response and conscious listening begins. If the orienting response is triggered, the person begins to decide "Is this new thing safe?" If the sound is familiar and matches a known sound, the brain may decide to filter out the sound unless it is important to the situation. This filtering is not always successful, even for the most functional adults, which is why some of us struggle in open-plan office spaces.

The orienting response may trigger neural connections from the midbrain to centers that control breathing, heart rate and other involuntary muscle contractions as the body prepares to react to the sound. Muscles at the core of the body or the neck may contract in preparation for physical response. Our bodies may rotate around our core to turn to face the source of the sound for further identification.

This is where a child's process of attention and habituation can break down. For children who have trouble building a strong database of sound during early development, many sounds trigger the orienting response when they should not. The impulse to attend and look to the source of sound is beyond their conscious control; their brains are not matching sounds with database files at a lower level of consciousness. When an incoming piece of sound information isn't accurately matched to an existing representation in the brain, then there is a "sensory mismatch", and the sound will rise to the level of consciousness. Therefore, whether or not a new piece of information invades a child's attention isn't a "choice", their lower-brain centers have already decided they need to redirect their attention to the new sound.

While the triggering of attention takes place in the midbrain, the next level of sensory processing of sound, takes place in the forebrain. Here the neural impulses created by the sound begin to be shunted to the necessary parts of the brain for processing. Does the information need to go to the auditory cortex for speech processing? What about the visual reception centers, for matching a sound with an image? Are there emotions involved in this sound information, such as in a song? In this case, the neural connections to the limbic system, our emotional center, will be activated. The limbic system

Catching Other's Emotions

When a piece of sound information also carries emotional content or special meaning for us, it is much more likely to form a memory as the limbic system becomes involved. As an example, think of a teacher whose lessons you remember compared with one you don't. Did the memorable teacher have enthusiasm for her subject? Did she convey this through tone of voice and pitch variation, or was her voice monotone? Did you already have a distinct interest in the subject, or was her excitement a bit contagious? Chances are she was stimulating your emotional center either through your own inherent interest in the subject or through social contagion (you caught your teacher's enthusiasm), and therefore your brain remembered the information more readily. This is why being able to hear the emotional content in speech delivered through changes in vocal pitch and harmonics (which we will explore in a later chapter) can be very important in learning and information retention.

also houses the hippocampus and amygdala, which are intimately involved in forming memories. Connecting the sound to all these important centers may be happening simultaneously.

Finally, the auditory cortex of the brain in the cerebrum receives the information, perhaps naming the sound and comparing it to past experience. "Is that Beethoven's 5th symphony? Yes, I've heard it before." The processing of this information may also involve the frontal cortex, where higher level decisions are made as we prepare to respond to a sound though further action. The visual cortex, in the back of the cerebrum may need to become involved, such as when we learned the alphabet. We needed to see the letter "A" to associate it repeatedly with the /a/ and /ah/ sounds.

When a baby is born, the neural connections from the inner ear to the brainstem are fully developed, but the connections to higher brain functions, such as the language centers if the brain, still need to be made. A child makes and strengthens these connections many, many times each day. There is research-based evidence for the idea of a database of sound. It has been proven that newborns already recognize voices in their environment as familiar, that certain combinations of sounds stimulate specific neural areas within the brain (an indication that a database file is being accessed within the brain), and that sounds with the same spectral (frequency-family) qualities become grouped together by the brain. But these specific neural connections become tenuous, or may not be formed at all, if the information with which they are created is not consistent. If there is an interruption to this development or an alteration in how sounds are perceived by the brain, a child's brain might "misfile" auditory information in their database.

Perhaps a sound that *should* be familiar may not be recognized in the child's sound database because it has been "misfiled." When that sound was initially encountered, it may have created a "new file" in the database. But, if subsequent encounters with that sound were not interpreted as the exact same, then it would not be matched up by the brain as a *recurring* sound. Therefore, every time that sound is encountered, it will register as different and novel, and therefore draw a child's attention more than it should.

For some children, an unfamiliar sound could create a stress response. Science writer Florence Williams discusses in her book *The Nature Fix*, that it is "only after [unrecognized] sound signals wash through our limbic brains that the frontal cortex gets to weigh in, for example interpreting the big rumble was a familiar DC-10 [airplane], not a marauding lion. In the microseconds in between, though, a stress response has already begun" (p. 90).

Conversely, a lack of correct files in the brain's sound database means that there are fewer points of reference for new learning. When too many sounds get misfiled in the brain, a child doesn't experience the repetition needed to build new skills based on experience. In this situation, the child's brain may become over-whelmed trying to file *every* sound as new and potentially useful, and resultantly close out attention to *any* auditory stimuli. Instead of having constantly divided attention, these children can focus intently on one thing and shut the rest of the world out. I have seen both types of children in my practice.

The Process in Reverse

Children who may have withdrawn from the overwhelming nature of their auditory world are able to shut out sounds because there are nerves that run in both directions. Neurons bring information from the ear to the brainstem to *and* from the brainstem to the ear (these are known as **efferent nerves**). The neural impulses going to the ear act to dampen sounds we don't want to hear by neurologically inhibiting the sound-receptor cells in our ear from firing. The two-way nature of our auditory nerves is important to us functionally, allowing us to isolate, locate, and habituate to noise around us. However, when listening is dampened because the brain is over-whelmed, this might create dysfunction. Blocked neural impulses can't allow new information in. In situations in which a child's brain has begun to dampen neural impulses that *should* be getting through, neural connections weaken when they should be strengthening. It is possible that a child's ability to filter out salient noises in the environment may become so strong as to inhibit their ability to respond to sound.

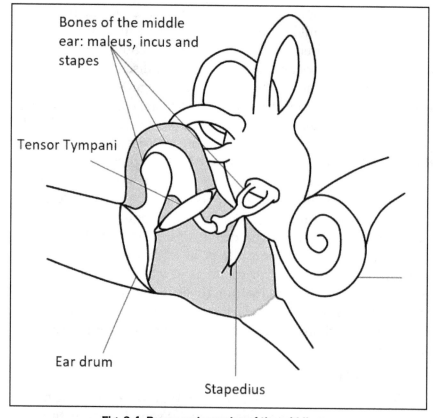

Fig. 3-4: Bones and muscles of the middle ear.

The neurons that travel from the brainstem to the ear, also control tiny muscles in the middle ear. Subconscious, reflex reactions control these muscles to serve two functions: to protect our hearing from overly-loud sounds and to help us better hear sounds that are important, despite competing noise. The two muscles of the middle ear that are controlled thusly are the **tensor tympani** muscle and the **stapedius** muscle.

The tensor tympani muscle attaches to the malleus, one of the three bones that transmit vibration of sound waves from our ear drum, also called the tympanic membrane (see Fig. 3-4). The malleus is the bone closest to the tympanic membrane and by pulling on it, the tensor tympani muscle can dampen the intensity of vibration of the membrane. This action helps preserve the integrity of the ear drum, and protects the very sensitive cells that interpret sound from overly-intense vibration. The tensor tympani helps protect our hearing against damage. Experimentally, you can activate the tensor tympani muscle at will by clenching your teeth, and hear its contraction's result on your hearing.

When a child is **<u>hypersensitive to sound</u>**, they will often cover their ears to sounds others can tolerate, or have significant behavioral problems in noisy environments. For these children, it may well be that the tensor tympani muscle is not doing its job. Because a functional tensor tympani protects the ear against damage, and damage to any part of the body creates pain signals in the brain, dysfunction in this muscle can create discomfort or pain for the child. Temple Grandin, a college professor and autistic person who explains how many autistic people feel about some sensations, describes her struggle with noise in her book *Thinking in Pictures*. She writes, "When I was little, loud noises were a problem, often feeling like a dentist's drill hitting a nerve" (p.63).

Another function of the tensor tympani muscle is to help us mitigate the sound of our own voices within our heads. As we will discuss later, bone-conducted sound is more intense and travels faster than air-conducted sound. The sound of our own voice is conducted through the tissues of our body (particularly effectively through our bones) from our vocal cords. When we speak, there is a neural reaction that activates the tensor tympani so that we don't hear our own voice twice—once intensely and immediately through bone-conduction, and again a millisecond later as air-conducted

---

The Face Expresses Emotions

When a child with Down Syndrome, who characteristically have low overall muscle tone and particularly low facial muscle tone, comes to my clinic, one of my favorite things to observe is the child's facial changes, possibly as a result of auditory therapy. Over the course of some months, the child's tongue might naturally retract into his mouth and his facial tone will increase. He'll begin to look older and more refined; more at home in his face and body and more ready to connect with others.

---

sound. A child with a dysfunction of the tensor tympani muscle may hear their own voice so intensely that they speak too quietly, or not make vocal noises at all.

Other efferent nerves help control the stapedius muscle of the middle ear (see Fig. 3-4). The stapedius muscle helps control what auditory pioneer Paul Madaule calls our "auditory zoom"; the ability to filter out background sounds to selectively focus on the frequency range our brain feels is relevant. When you listen to a friend's story in a crowded, noisy restaurant, your auditory zoom helps the bones in your ear vibrate more intensely in the frequency range of your friend's voice. And thus, *not* vibrate at the lower-pitched frequencies of mechanical noises or more distant conversations. Undesirable sound waves are hitting your ear drum simultaneously with the waves of sounds you *do* want to hear. In order to better hear the salient sounds (often the frequency ranges involved in speech), the bones of the middle ear should vibrate in the frequencies that transmit those sounds. This is achieved by the contraction of the *stapedius* muscle, which connects to the stapes, the last bone in the three-bone chain leading from the eardrum to the cochlea. The stapedius contracts to narrow the range of vibration in which the desired sound falls.

The stapedius muscle also helps the ear zoom in on the complex tones in the human voice that **communicate emotion**. Interestingly, the cranial nerve that carries information to and from the stapedius muscle, the Facial nerve, also innervates the muscles of the face that *express* emotion. A maxim posited by the granddaddy of auditory therapy, Alfred Tomatis, is that "the voice only reproduces those tones which the ear is likely to hear." This may help to explain why children with auditory processing problems and/or autism have flat speech with little vocal tone variation and few facial expressions. If they have a stapedius muscle that is not helping to transmit the human voice in all its complexity, then they are not hearing the subtleties of vocal expression (the tenderness, or confusion, or sarcasm), only the content. Since they can't hear the emotion in others' voices, they may not be able to reproduce those emotions communicatively.

Both the tensor tympani and the stapedius muscle move miniscule, feather-light bones in the middle ear. The middle ear is an enclosed space where the fluid from an ear infection can build up, thicken, and increase pressure behind the ear drum. For children who have had multiple ear infections or fluid build-up (perhaps from repeated allergies), these muscles may be too poorly calibrated to respond correctly to sound. Imagine that your arm was trying to learn to lift a glass of water to your mouth, and you had no way of knowing how full or heavy the glass was. Each time you started to lift the glass, you couldn't know how much force to use to lift it smoothly and effectively. You would have to go very slowly each time to avoid spilling the water. In this situation, the muscles of your arm are not be properly calibrated to automatically use the right amount of force. For children with middle ear issues, the muscles of the ear have trouble learning the correct force to use to

---

A Surgical Intervention to Explore

Pressure Equalization tubes are placed in the tympanic membrane (ear drum) of the ear, allowing excess fluid to drain from the middle ear. This keeps the pressure of the middle ear more constant, although the viscosity of the fluid in the middle ear (how thick or thin it is) can vary with further infections, allergies, colds, etc. It has been my experience that some children make improvements in motor and speech skills after PE tubes are placed. Some otolaryngologists (ENTs) are hesitant to place **PE tubes** unless a threshold of a certain number of ear infections per year has been met. If your child has had a number of ear infections, frequent colds or consistent respiratory allergies, you may want to visit the idea of PE tube placement with your child's doctor.

control the bones, as the pressure and viscosity of the fluid in the middle ear changes from day to day. This may cause delayed sound processing and possibly be related to slowness in speech processing for children whose hearing acuity is completely normal.

It is possible that, for a child with variable pressure behind their ear drum, the same noise might sound different from day to day. Returning to the idea of a sound database, a repeated sound might get misfiled in the brain's sound database as a novel sound each time. It may not become associated with the appropriate response from the child, or it may always seem like a new sound. The learning that *should* result from hearing a sound repeatedly may not occur for that child.

Auditory Development and the Root of Communication

In the womb, the inner ear houses the first sensory systems in the body to become fully-myelinated and therefore to receive and transmit accurate sensory input. A newborn baby's vision is blurry and inaccurate, and difficult to direct. The sense of touch evolves throughout childhood, as an accurate brain-map of a child's ever-changing body must develop through daily, repeated contact with people and things. But the cochleae and vestibulae (the plural of cochlea and vestibulum; remember that everyone has two) have complete function and accurate connections with the brainstem

---

Listening Before Birth

The tensor tympani muscle protects us from hearing our own voices too loudly and damaging our hearing when we speak, since bone-conducted sound is so much louder. During development in utero, a baby begins to run out of space in the womb around six months' gestation. The baby's head begins to contact the mother's ribs or pelvis or spine. This is a chance for the baby to start to develop the tensor tympani muscle, blocking bone-conducted sound. Also, the stapedius muscle begins to allow the ear to focus on specific frequencies, like those of mom's voice. Knowing these muscles get quite a workout before birth means that babies who are in the breech position, born prematurely, or were exposed to toxic chemicals (i.e., drugs and alcohol) in the womb, may not have had a chance to experience this crucial phase of development.

while still in the womb. Consider the Moro, or startle, reflex with which babies are born. That reflex is activated by a loud sound or by rapidly lowering a newborn from a height. A baby won't respond in such an immediate, protective way by seeing something, even a bright light, or by touching something unexpectedly. But hearing and movement are sensed accurately, perceiving possible dangers, from the moment of birth.

Because the auditory system is fully developed in the womb, it is beginning to help the child interpret the world even before birth. One of the primary auditory skills developed *in utero* is learning the difference between foreground and background noise. The world inside a mother's womb is loud, with low-frequency noises of mother's blood rushing and heart beating and digestion. Early in gestation, the mother's voice and other outside sounds travel though tissues and amniotic fluid, and may be difficult for the fetus to distinguish from background sounds. However, around the sixth month of gestation, the fetus typically reaches a size in which his head makes periodic contact with the mother's spine or pelvic bones. Sound travels much more easily and loudly through Mom's bones than through amniotic fluid, so the higher-pitched sounds of the mother's voice begin to come into auditory focus.

This is the beginning of auditory zoom, our ears' ability to home

---

Learning Before Birth

Humans aren't the only species that "practice" skills before birth. One of my favorite illustrations of this is a story I once heard about the humble chicken. Chicks hatch, and within moments begin pecking the ground, ostensibly for food. Hens don't show their newborn chicks how to do this, or what "food" looks like to a chicken, or where it is located. How do new chicks know what to do then? A scientist in China discovered that if you coat a chicken egg in petroleum jelly, you can study the chick inside without disturbing it. At a certain point during incubation, a chick runs out of room to grow in the shell and begins to curl up upon itself. Its head comes in contact with its chest. Inside its chest, its heart is beating many times per minute, and with each beat, the chick's head goes up and down in a pecking motion. Therefore, the chick is continuing to perform the movement he learned in the shell, pecking, immediately after birth.

in on the frequency the brain would like to hear. Not only is this repeated activity in the womb a chance for baby to get primed to tune into *Mom's* voice after birth, but to all voices. Voices in the environment *should* attract a child's attention so that communication and socialization can develop. This skill is so important that we all get a few months to practice it before we have to interact with the world.

After developing auditory zoom and attention to voice in the womb, we begin to layer new skills on top of this knowledge upon our arrival in the outside world. Sound becomes much more connected with movement. We learn to control our eyes to send our gaze in the direction of Mom's voice. We learn about object-permanence, the idea that something we cannot see still exists, because we hear Dad's voice even when we can't see him. Our neck and core muscles develop as we turn toward a sound. Locating sound sources helps infants develop accurate head-and-neck movements, strengthens core muscles and encourages visual scanning of the environment to develop accurate eye muscle movement.

We are born with recognition of vocal sounds as relevant and alerting, and this initiates communication, and also develops the requisite eye- and neck-muscle motor control that go along with communication. This process might be short-circuited for people with autism. Both Naoki Higashida, a young man with autism, and Therese Joliffe, a woman with autism, say that they **don't always realize a nearby person is speaking**, and whether that person is addressing them. Joliffe explains in her article "Autism: A personal account" that her ear does not isolate voices in the environment easily, and she often loses the first few words of what someone is saying to her because it takes longer for her to realize someone *is* speaking, and to her.

Building a Sound Database of Where and What

In addition to being the root of learning about communication and social connection, the auditory sense is a large part of the foundation on which understanding the physical world is built. Babies not only receive sounds *from* the world, they generate them as well. Cooing and babbling, in addition to being adorable, has always been thought to be babies' "practice" at communicating with other people. But what if babies coo and babble to communicate with *themselves*—to inform themselves about the world around them?

Babies' brains use the sounds bouncing back to them from their own vocal noises to help establish visual depth perception and to begin to make predictions about the qualities of objects. In illustration: imagine a 3-month-old baby placed on her belly on soft carpet. As she babbles, the sound is reflected from inches away; she confirms this distance with her hands and her eyes focus on her hands. Then her mother moves her to a linoleum floor. The quality of the sound has changed; she still confirms the distance with her hands, but she begins to build a database of how different surfaces sound, look and feel.

As this same baby begins to sit around the sixth month, she continues to respond to sounds in the environment and sounds bouncing back to her from her babbling. Now she incorporates head, neck, and core rotation to choose where her eyes and ears are directed in her environment. As sounds take variable time to bounce back to her from different distances, she learns to control the convergence of her eyes on objects both near and far, and her **visual depth perception** becomes more finely-tuned. As she gains a better understanding of depth and distance, she begins to want things outside her immediate reach, things that are close enough to *try* to get to. Using her understanding of where the ground is underneath her and how her body reacts to it, she begins to roll, scoot, crawl, and eventually, walk to what she wants.

While many people know the sequence of physical development—the order of development of physical skills—this understanding of everything our auditory sense tells us might explain the *motivation* for movement and the *reason* one wants to develop motor skills. For example, why does a baby reach for an object near them, but just out of reach? This is often the impetus for a baby's first roll or scoot. How do they know that rattle is attainable, while other things in their visual world are too far away? Is it possible that this "guess" that something is attainable is initially auditorily-based?

Learning builds upon itself in increments, and ocular-motor skills and body-motor skills likely develop on knowledge with which the child already has experience. Auditory function is a primary root of the child's developing database of knowledge. When we look at learning in this way, it is easier to understand that prematurity, breech birth, multiple ear infections or allergies may significantly impact a child's motor and cognitive development down the line. Yet, when a child is delayed in motor or cognitive skills, they are often provided therapy that does not address the auditory sense.

Addressing Auditory Function in Therapy

One of auditory therapy's many effects might be understood better by considering the stapedius muscle. If we were to rehabilitate any muscle in the body, we would expect to have exercises that strengthen and refine the use of that muscle. Recall from earlier, that if the stapedius is not functioning optimally, a child will have trouble processing speech, both drawing it out of background noise and processing its meaning through emotional content. Because stapedius function, and therefore auditory filtering of sound, doesn't involve the higher "thinking" brain centers, a child's lack of attention when someone is speaking to them cannot be treated as effectively using cognitive methods. In other words, it is not as effective to try to *teach* a child to pay attention by consciously working on filtering and attending skills, than it is to exercise the stapedius muscle. When the stapedius muscle is more responsive and accurate, a child's brain more-readily recognizes the auditory cues for attention and filtering. Because this function is subconscious, we must help the ear learn to respond accurately to sound by allowing opportunities to strengthen and calibrate the stapedius muscle.

The passive appearance of participation in auditory therapy is actually a bit deceptive. Our ears are working behind the scenes to orient us, and re-orient us when the need arises, all day. The time spent participating in auditory therapy is an enhanced opportunity for a child's ears and their brain to strengthen those orienting neural connections, so the child can use those neurons functionally their headphones are NOT on. There are physical clues that can be observed when the sounds in the headphones are drawing a child's attention, and similarly when a child is actively filtering out the sounds to attend to a task. During therapy, the child is practicing the dance of habituation and attention that all of us perform all day, and this creates stronger neural connections for learning when the headphones come off.

For the curious, more specifics on the theory and practice of auditory therapy and the different types of auditory therapy that are available can be found in the appendix at the back of this book.

4   The Brain's HAL 9000

To understand how we attend to, hear, and potentially respond to sound, it might be helpful to begin at the end. The final steps in the listening process, before we perform any sort of response to an incoming sound, are recognition and categorization. Recognizing a sound often occurs through a visual confirmation of where the sound is coming from. This involves a complex neurological process of specific sound location, which we will explore later. For now, let's investigate how we recognize sounds as familiar; the idea of a "sound database" and how it develops.

Sounds we hear throughout our lives get "coded" by the brain. At the most simplistic level, a very consistent, very simple sound, such as the short "beep" from a child's toy gets its own file in the sound database. However, most sounds in our environment are much more complex: they may have sources that travel within our environment, like a car driving by, or they may be variants on the same type of sound, like different notes played by the same instrument. Imagine you are listening to an orchestra playing a symphony live for the first time. If your brain had to code every note from every instrument as unique and file it in your database, you'd have no brain-space left to enjoy the music! Luckily, your previous experience with music and your brain's natural propensity to categorize sensations into groups allows this experience to be filed under "music, orchestral, classical, Beethoven, 9th Symphony" and your brain is then free to let the music work its magic on you.

But how does this phenomenal achievement of the mind occur? Through early life, the brain codes different sounds and stores them. When a sound arrives with which there is a likely match, those two sounds get grouped together. The brain compares its previous experience to a new sound's duration, location, and **spectral** (frequency and tone) **qualities** to create "sound rules." From these sound rules, new information is categorized and even predicted. When an incoming sound does not match a file in the brain, or does not match what the brain had predicted based on experience, additional brain neurons are activated to help assess the new sound. This occurrence can be observed using brain-imaging techniques and is a very important tool in studying how the brain responds to sound. It is called **mismatch negativity** (MMN). In response to MMN, the brain recruits more neurons to compare this sound, that doesn't quite match, to what a person already knows.

When mismatch negativity does not occur, when we are listening to familiar sounds, our neural response to those sounds is actually dampened through a neural process called **stimulus-specific adaptation** (SSA). SSA is the process through which habituation to sound takes place. When a continuing sound is categorized as "known, not a threat and not relevant to the task at hand" by the brain, it sends an inhibitory signal to the ear essentially saying, "Hey neurons, stop firing. We don't need that information." Think about the air conditioning unit in your house cycling on while you're working. You might notice it, but then you don't hear it anymore, until it cycles off.

This SSA process can happen at the brainstem level, without conscious attention. When you are awake, you may notice the cycling of the air conditioning, but it rarely rises to the same level of consciousness while you are asleep. Your brain decides at a subconscious level that the sound is irrelevant to sleeping.

Brains build their sound databases by detecting these small changes in the environment, and possibly responding with SSA or MMN. As the database grows, the brain develops neural "representations" of the sounds it encounters; a specific set of neurons that fire when they hear that sound. The brain then groups those representations into categories. Throughout development, the SSAs happen more often, and the MMNs are only activated if the sound is novel or particularly relevant to the task at hand. As our database grows larger and we begin to have greater autonomous control over our attention and concentration. For this development to occur, neurological response to sound in the environment must be consistent, based on sound information the brain has deemed "dependable." If the ears or their connections are compromised due to disease or damage, then this essential chain of events could be compromised as well, and attention and concentration to relevant stimuli may be thrown out of whack.

What's in the Database

In the previous chapter, the idea of a sound/depth perception database was introduced. But the brain creates sound connections for all sorts of sensory information, adding those connections to various files. There are sound/spectral-family connections that help us categorically recognize sounds that we have never encountered but are similar to other sounds we have. Sound/object files are created when incredibly precise eye movements find the source of a sound, creating a visual representation of which object made which sound. The sound/thalamus connection in the brain helps us create files for things without a physical manifestation, like an idea, such as a song, or an emotion, such as the "upset and angry" tone of voice. Finally, the brain has files for sound/time connections, which we will explore as a key component of verbal communication, social interaction and physical movement.

As I write this, a truck has rumbled by on our street. We live in a pretty quiet neighborhood, so the sound was caught by my ears as being different, a bit louder than cars driving by at intervals. But how did I know it was a truck, and not another car, or an airplane, or some alien spaceship that decided my neighborhood was ripe for invasion? Did it sound exactly like every other truck that I had ever encountered? Well, no. Because different engines have different sound signatures, different tires sound differently on different surfaces, different levels of sound as the truck drives past at different speeds, etc. no two trucks sound exactly the same. So, how did I know?

Every sound in an environment has a range of amplitudes and phases that is unique to that sound. We tend to think of sounds as simple waves, issuing from one point in space in a nice rhythmic fashion. However, all naturally-occurring sounds are *combinations* of many waves of varying amplitudes (intensities) and phases (frequencies). Although no two trucks sound alike, most have similar pitches that overlap into the complex "truck" sound.

Our brains produce a neurological sound/spectral-family analysis of every sound because our cochleae act like tiny filters, finding all the phases and amplitudes contained within a sound, but continuing to group them together as the same sound, mostly based on time of arrival to the ear. The brain combines this spectral analysis with other information about the sound into its database files for a given sound. Not just the spectrum of the sound, but it's timing relative to the expected environment, duration, location, travel, and volume. If the sound outside my house had been of the same spectrum as my file for "truck", but been a shorter duration, louder, or not travelled across my field of hearing, I'd likely have to go to the window to see what's going on. Our ears develop sound groups that are associated with "truck rumble", or "baby crying", or "door slamming." Consequently, I don't have to look out my window to know that a truck is rumbling past my house.

Harmonics Create Meaning

How does a child come to know that the noise they are hearing in their environment is a human voice and not some other sound, like a toy or music? One way is through the priming the baby's brain receives in utero, by hearing his mother's voice (which we explored in a previous chapter). But how does the child come to realize that other people use these sounds to communicate thoughts and ideas, and not just make random noises with their mouths? How do babies begin to solve the problem that infant-development researchers Alison Gopnik, Andrew Meltzoff and Patricia Kuhl called the "Language Problem"? One way is through sound localization; the child hears a noise and locates the source of the sound as another person, the physics of which we'll get into later. However, other important factors at play in language and communication are **harmonics** and **pitch relativity**.

When you listen to the note 'A' on the musical scale, a pitch of 440 Hz, how do you know if the note is being played on a violin, a flute or being sung? The answer is harmonics. That 'A' note makes sound waves that occur at 440 cycles per second, but those sound waves are not simply an up-and-down wave shape. They are a combination of many frequencies in various concentrations, which reinforce or counter each other, so that the combined effect is the frequency of 440 Hz. It's the variation and the number of different frequencies, the harmonics, creating the *pitch* of 440 Hz that allow

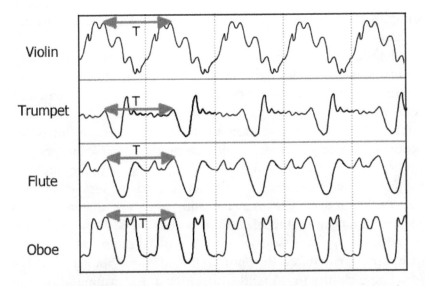

Fig. 4-1: Harmonic images of instruments playing the same note

our ear to distinguish between violin, trumpet, oboe, flute or anything else that can produce that pitch. In the illustration above, you can see that each instrument is producing a pitch at the same wave-length, T, but it is a combination of waves creating different shapes across this interval that gives them a different sound.

In Fig. 4-1, you can see that the wavelengths from crest to crest at the same interval "T", meaning they are the same pitch, but the wave shapes differences create the differences between instruments that your ear perceives.

Harmonics help explain why people's voices sound different from one another. To a large extent, the variation in harmonics and pitch in our voice is what <u>communicates our thoughts</u>, not necessarily the words that compose what we say. If you ask your kids to get ready to leave the house, you can communicate this verbally any number of ways; "Get your shoes on", "Let's go in five minutes", "We have to head to the store." What gets their attention, and really tells them to move, is the amount of urgency in your voice. And that is created through harmonics. More important information, with greater emotional content, is delivered with more higher-pitched harmonics. Think about saying, "Come on, let's move!" versus "I think we'll have steak for dinner tonight." Even if you don't alter the volume or pitch of your voice, the nature of what you say in these two examples feels different, and that difference is delivered through harmonics.

If a child's ear and brain are not attuned to hear the emotional differences in speech through harmonics, learning language becomes an exercise in rote memorization of how words sound and matching them with their meanings. This is why many children with communication disorders, even those that have some functional speech, continue to struggle with communication concepts like humor, empathy and warnings. If they cannot **perceive the emotions** in others, young children won't be able to express their own nuances of emotion. They may continue to only be able to express the basic emotions of anger, happiness or sadness. They don't hear the subtle change in person's voice when they become satisfied (but not happy), or irritated (but not angry), or disappointed (but not sad). These children also tend to have trouble **grasping idioms or sarcasm** well after their peers have developed these abilities, and that can limit their opportunities for social engagement with friends.

Grandin describes herself as having very little emotional range; "I definitely do have [emotions], but they are more like the emotions of a child than an adult... [emotional] nuances are still incomprehensible to me" (p.89). People with autism and other auditory processing problems may be missing the emotional content of speech and therefore a huge part of learning about the world. Hearing emotional components of communication allows them to develop sympathy with others and come to understand that individuals can feel differently about the same events or objects. For example, to hear satisfaction in another's voice (and see it in their face) as they bite into chocolate helps a child begin to understand that other people may like chocolate, even if the child does not.

Lower-Pitched Speakers

So, if an increase in higher-pitched sounds in our voices indicates emotionally-charged content in our speech, why doesn't a deep-voiced man start to sound like a soprano when he's emotionally excited? As more higher-pitched harmonics enter into speech sounds, they are counter-balanced by more lower-pitched harmonics as well. It's the big gap between high and low frequencies that create the same pitch that catch the attention or our ears and minds, not necessarily a rise in sound pitch.

The other component that that falls outside of one's choice of words, but is also key to delivering the meaning behind our communication is pitch relativity. This distinction is easiest to observe in hearing yourself ask a question. When communicating a question, our voice naturally goes up in pitch to communicate the lack of certainty about what we are asking. Ask someone, "Did you want steak for dinner?" versus saying, "We are having steak for dinner" and you'll hear the difference clearly.

It doesn't matter if the person speaking has a high- or a low-pitched voice. It's the change in pitch across the phrase or sentence that communicates the meaning, not the absolute pitch of each word or sound. Babies trying to figure out the meaning of language begin by recognizing patterns of pitch relativity. This is why we naturally speak to babies with exaggerated ups and downs in our speech patterns. They are learning to recognize inflections in our speech that carry meaning, and the words attached to those meanings will come later.

In his class "Music and the Brain", psychology professor Aniruddh Patel tells us that humans are the only species that has an ability to take a relative pitch sequence, like a melody, move it up or down a musical scale, and still recognize it as the same set of sounds. If you heard a melody and then heard the same melody played in the next lower octave, you would still recognize the two melodies as the same song. Birds can make beautiful and sometimes very complicated melodies, but they are unable to recreate or recognize their species song if the pitch is altered, but it's timing and sequencing are not. That's why you cannot tell one robin's song from another; they all sing the same notes the same way. And if you translated the robin's song down one octave, say by playing back a modified recording, the robin would not recognize it as a robin's song.

This is part of the explanation as to why humans can communicate with such complex language, uniquely among all animals. We can communicate not just by shaping our mouths into different sounds, but by intoning our speech with emotional content through harmonics and pitch variation that conveys rich meanings across a huge spectrum of ideas. When you reflect on how complicated human speech is and how much the ear and brain must process in each individual moment of sound information, it becomes easier to see how any auditory dysfunction would not only impact language and speech development but also behavior and cognitive processes. This is why addressing the cascading effects of an inner ear problem by addressing the resulting behavior or deficit, without addressing what has gone wrong within the ear and its neural connections, is so much more difficult, time-consuming and frustrating, and not as effective.

Our Ears Develop Our Eyes

In the previous chapter, the idea of depth-perception development through sound-wave reflection was explored through the example of a baby lying on the floor. Remember that the sound bouncing from the baby's mouth to the carpet and back again sounded different than when the baby was lying on linoleum? Different surfaces have different sound-reflections. As babies interact with their world, listening and touching, they add sound/texture combinations to their sound database. They also couple these sensations with how a surface looks; how light bounces off it and if the surface is three-dimensional. These connections in their database help their nervous system prepare itself for the upcoming tactile sensation of touching the surface.

The idea of sound/texture database finds logical evidence in the fact that one of the first stops for a sound's neural impulse once it leave the ear is the **dorsal cochlear nucleus,** located in the brainstem, which also receives sensory input from receptors in the skin. This could be the first place these two streams of sensation meet to travel to their database file in the brain.

A well-developed sight/sound/touch database can limit the number of unexpected, and perhaps unpleasant, **tactile experiences** a child has as they explore the world around them. Have you ever reached out to touch a surface you thought would be smooth and solid because it was glossy and immobile, and it turned out to be squishy and feel a little wet? You probably were surprised, and maybe even a little grossed-out, as you pulled your hand back. Can you imagine if your whole day was filled with unpleasant surprises like this one?

That may have been the case for my little friend Tyler. Tyler was three-years-old, but short for his size after being born prematurely and having multiple health issues leading to multiple hospitalizations in his young life. Although his physical skills were not well-coordinated, he was able to walk with a walker (which he discarded as therapy continued) and he could speak, although his voice was monotone and his emotional expression was limited (but would also improve during therapy). He was hesitant and anxious about most things, but his limited sound/sight/touch database was demonstrated for me the first time he encountered a Koosh ball. You might remember Koosh balls, as they were popular for quite a while in the 1990s. They are balls meant to be thrown and caught, or just touched, for fun. They are not round but have many rubbery, hair-like projections, making them a unique tactile sensation. But for Tyler, different was *not* fun. The movement of the hairs of the ball in response to his touch was unexpected and very upsetting to him. He had no sound file for the way this thing behaved, and its movement may have even been stimulating to lower brain centers that control the fight-or-flight response, as it responded to touch with quasi-lifelike movement. No way was he touching that ball! But as we worked on his ability to use sound to predict textures, the Koosh ball and other new surfaces became less threatening.

It's also noteworthy that Tyler was a very **picky eater**. If a child doesn't know, based on their sound-database of experiences, what something might feel like to touch with their hands, they are most likely not going to be enthusiastic about putting it in their mouths. Putting an unidentifiable object in one's mouth is threatening for a few reasons. Breathing also occurs through the mouth, and being able to coordinate the chew-swallow-breathe sequence may already be challenging for the child. Also, a child can't visually monitor the interaction of his mouth with the object to make sure everything is OK. While eating aversions can seem arbitrary and irrational, they might begin to make sense when viewed through the eyes of a child for whom all the necessary information about a situation is not available, causing them to feel threatened. Eating aversions are complex issues and they can have multiple roots, but I rarely see this auditory aspect of eating problems addressed in traditional therapy.

Making Sound Memories

The **hippocampi** (plural of hippocampus, every brain has two) play a key role in forming emotions, creating memories and also contributes to the control of the autonomic nervous system, which controls our fight-or-flight responses. We can sometimes observe the emotional effect of sound on ourselves; an unexpected noise creating a moment of fear or a beautiful piece of music creating an emotional response. Both of these scenarios may call for a response from us, which is why the **amygdala** is also involved in the process. The amygdala is the brain's center for processing emotions and their contribution to decision-making.

For the hippocampus to participate and form memories based on sound, the sound must be emotionally or situationally relevant to the hearer. In a 2006 study on perceptual learning by Polley et al., adult rats did not create new neural connections unless a sound was behaviorally-relevant. If they were expected to incorporate the sound into their decision-making process (such as using sound to find their way through a maze to food), then that sound formed new memory for them. If the sound was not linked to some behavioral expectation, then the neural response in their brain did not indicate a memory of the sound when it was presented again. It may be that, in the human brain, new neural patterns are created only if sounds have emotional meaning or are relevant to function. In other words, for a person to create a new "sound file" in the database, the sound must carry some meaning; be it emotional or relevant to function.

Time and the Database

Just as there are database files for ideas and objects affiliated with sounds and words, there are database files associated with things that are auditory, but are *not* sounds. Namely, spaces without sound and spaces between sounds. These pauses in sound carry a great many meanings for the brain, and thus the brain creates files so it can remember the timing, duration and space between sounds. In an elegantly-designed experiment by Winkler et al. (2009), measurable mismatch negativity was created in a newborn's brain when the expected downbeat in a rhythmic structure is *not* played. In other words, when listening to a rhythm, a newborn creates a sound-time file for that rhythm, and if the rhythm violates the rhythmically-established sound "rules" (such as an overly-long pause between beats), the infant brain has a moment of neural pique in which it wonders what the deal is.

This database of sound and time is formed very early on, and it helps the brain develop an **understanding of time** that influences a range of functions: physical responses, coordination, socially appropriate behavior, emotional responses, and the development of a vocabulary centered around time concepts. In the development of an understanding of time, listening is primary among the senses because it is the only sensory input in which *time is an essential component* for correct sensory interpretation. When we use any of our senses, the transmission of neural impulses requires a very short span of time, but listening requires those neural impulses to be put into the context of what came before and after to be interpreted correctly. One hears words, songs and environmental sounds across a span of time. The meaning of each individual sound is only understood within the context of the sounds that come before and after. There are specific neurons in the brain to help determine the context of any sound. Is a single sound a note in a song? What kind of song; a sad one, a march? Is it part of a word or sentence? How long is the pitch held? Where did the sound come from?

In addition to context, two important time-related aspects of interpreting sound are understanding the amount of time sounds take to occur, and understanding the amount of time between sounds. As an infant's brain builds a database of spatial and spectral files, it also constructs a time-sound database, beginning to develop rudimentary concepts of time by noticing the spaces between sounds in daily rhythms. In the heartbeat of the mother in the womb, in the songs we use to soothe babies, and in the cadence of a nursery rhyme, a child is surrounded by rhythm all day. Infant-development researchers Maurer and Maurer state that a child's brain is capable of measuring the space between sounds down to $1/50^{th}$ of a second.

Rhythm is how the brain teaches itself about time. The concept of time is a particularly difficult one to "teach" someone at a cognitive level. You can't physically point to a second or a minute to define them for someone who doesn't understand. A person learning about time must be able to feel time passing, and measure it in discreet segments.

To understand how the brain uses spaces in rhythms, consider this example: You are watching a metronome; the kind with the weighted arm that swings from side-to-side. If the metronome is *not* making its accompanying ticking sound, and you sit for about five minutes watching it, you might have trouble knowing that five, and not ten, minutes have passed. However, if the sound is on, you are likely to be much more accurate in your assessment of how much time has passed. With the sound turned on, your brain measures the spaces between the ticks and knows about how much time has passed. Without the sound you might become mesmerized and lose track of time. A person's brain uses the space between sounds to create a more accurate sense of time.

I believe that children with autism can become mesmerized easily because of the lack of internalized understanding of time passage. Because they may have no, or a very tenuous, anchor to time concepts, they can spend what others would consider a very long time experiencing the same sensation repeatedly. Temple Grandin refers to this very specifically in her book, *Thinking in Pictures*. "When left alone, I would often space out and become hypnotized." Grandin doesn't relate this phenomenon to a lack of understanding of time, however, perhaps because she wouldn't recognize the concept of time awareness as innate to neurotypical people.

Other Functions of Time

The small spaces between sounds that create rhythm are the beginning of the brain's understanding of time. Spans of time are also important as a child learns to communicate with others. Verbal communication is extremely dependent on time as a component of meaning. Think about this sentence: "I didn't want her to take the money." What might this sentence mean? Well, depending on the vocal stress on a given word, lots of things. Vocal stress is most noticeably communicated through the amount of time applied a given word in comparison to the rest of the sentence.

- *I* didn't want her to take the money.

- I *didn't* want her to take the money.

- I didn't *want* her to take the money.

- I didn't want *her* to take the money.

- I didn't want her to take *the money*.

As important as time and rhythm are in communicating a person's meaning, spaces in time between words also carry significant **meaning during speech**. Human beings do something astonishing when we communicate, something no other species does. In a mature conversation between peers, there is an infinitesimal space in one person's speech in which it is socially appropriate for the other person to interject or begin speaking. It takes less than a second, but the functional brain recognizes this pause accurately. And researchers have found that it happens across all cultures, in any language.

The brain that measures pauses incorrectly will have difficulty communicating; committing social faux pas, or not realizing when they don't have all of the information a person is trying to communicate. If a child does not develop the natural ability to recognize that pauses communicate the completion of a thought, then they might not realize when they have not heard the entire idea. For example, a teacher if trying to correct a child's behavior with the following sentence, "When we play with others, it is not OK to take their toys without asking." There is a lot of sequencing and quite a long train of thought for a child to follow. And constructing the meaning of the sentence in a child's brain can be downright impossible if their basic sense of timing doesn't let them follow the sentence in its entirety.

Pauses within speech can also have other meanings as well. Imagine you ask your child if they have taken something that belongs to you. If they answer too quickly or pause too long before answering, your brain is likely to analyze their response as untruthful. If you ask someone how their day was, and they pause before responding, "Fine", are they really fine? This subtlety in receptive communication takes experience (and database files) to develop, but it can help to explain while children tend to be more gullible and guileless than adults, why sarcasm may be beyond their grasp, and why comedic timing develops only as children mature. The ability to distinguish a person's actual meaning when their words do not match their actions requires refined levels of processing, but it becomes impossible to build those abilities without an accurate sense of time.

Science demonstrates that, in the functional human brain, sounds of durations of up to three seconds are perceived as a whole, but after three seconds, structures of the brain involved in short-term, working memory must be involved. If the construct of time is poorly perceived or the sequencing of sounds by the brain is impaired, then the working memory of the brain may not engage when necessary. This may help to explain why a child can remember that you told them to clean up his room, but not that you told him to pick up his room *and* take the trash out. It took you more than three seconds to say it.

Many children I see in the clinic have verbal skills that allow them to express simple ideas, such as "I want a cookie", but at older ages, like seven and eight, their academic development becomes delayed because they are unable to build conceptual ideas about what they learn. They are processing the sounds that are received, but not comprehending the whole in manageable "chunks" of information. This may be because the timing mechanism in their brain is not allowing them to engage their working memory at the correct time, and consequently they stay engaged in immediate reception of sound. They become unable to recognize and package discreet pieces of information for filing in their database. If a child can use **working memory** to build separate "chunks" of auditory information into a cohesive whole, learning concepts becomes easier.

In his remarkable book *Felt Time*, German psychologist Marc Wittman states that a well-developed sense of time can also act as a warning system for our brain; there can be a sensory mismatch when something is "taking too long" that alerts us that trouble could be afoot. When the timer on the stove doesn't sound after the expected amount of time, you might realize you forgot to set it. The brain continues to track time even in sleep; when we get enough sleep, but forget to set our alarm, we may oversleep by a few minutes. But we are likely to snap awake very near the time we were meant to get out of bed.

As a child develops, they learn to associate words with concepts of time, and this can help tremendously in establishing **socially-appropriate behaviors**. They learn that "a minute" is about the length of a simple song, and that "later" means a much large span of time. This can be helpful when they would like a glass of juice, and an adult responds with, "In a minute" while they head to the kitchen for the juice, versus "later" in which they might have to go to the store for the juice. The child now knows how long he must wait for juice and may decide a tantrum isn't worth it, especially if the juice is forthcoming.

This time-awareness can be a key component of helping children deal with behaviors such as impatience, anxiety, or attention. When a child has a concept of "tomorrow" versus "next year", adults can begin to allay children's concerns about the sequence of events in a day and what is coming in the future. If an understanding of socially-important spans of time is missing for a child, they might experience anxiety about the course of the future or uncertainty about what will be expected of them and when. Many of the families I begin working with can't mention upcoming vacations to their child, or they will have to endure endless daily questioning; "Do we go to Disney today? Do we go to Disney tomorrow? When do we go to Disney?..." Clinically, I know we have made progress in time-concepts when a child begins to correctly refer to "yesterday" and "tomorrow" in the proper sequence, or mention that they will see me again next week, not tomorrow. They are becoming more grounded in the sequence of their days and their understanding of time.

My buddy Paul helped me understand the impact that subtle auditory processing issues, like not having a well-developed sense of time, can have on behavior and function. At almost seven years of age, Paul had already gone through kindergarten twice, and his mother was worried that he would have to repeat first-grade as well if he wasn't better able to retain new information and participate in class. She was also frustrated by his multiple word mispronunciations and his inability to correct them no matter how many times she demonstrated the proper way to say a word. He also had problems finding the words he wanted to express himself. For example, in recounting a story he called a convertible an "outside car."

While Paul rarely got into trouble at school, when he did it was for not being able to keep his hands to himself, in a playful way, and for not following directions. Although he had tantrums when things did not go his way, he was never violent. He was what I would call "benevolently aggressive", poking his younger brother and the family dog to provoke them, but seemingly in the context of a game to which only he knew the rules—that is to say, it was never done with malice. His mom reported that during even short car rides, Paul would poke or pinch his brother and have very little remorse about making his brother upset.

Because of his speech problems and word-finding difficulties, I knew that auditory treatment would be the focus of our initial therapy. After two months of therapy, he was retaining information better and his behavior was better overall. Sometimes he was able to negotiate for what he needed instead of having a tantrum, indicating a new ability to follow the course of a conversation and understand the projection of ideas into the near future.

While he was less aggressive toward the family dog and his brother while at home, car rides were still an issue for his mother, as she couldn't monitor his behavior as closely while driving. So, what was going on during car rides? At the time, I really didn't know. However, as his auditory therapy progressed and we addressed rhythm and the spaces between sounds, some interesting changes developed. He began using words like "yesterday" and "tomorrow" with accuracy, meaning that broad concepts of time were beginning to make sense to him. As this sense of time became more refined, he was able to organize, and more importantly *reorganize*, his day in his head. If he was planning on coming home from school to go out to play, and instead his mother had to run to the grocery store before dinner, he was no longer thrown into a tailspin. He inherently knew how long a trip to the store would take, how long the afternoon before dinner was, and that he would have time to play outside before dinner.

Before these fine-tuned concepts of time were unavailable to Paul, he organized his day by events, "First we come home, then we play outside, then we have dinner." He couldn't conceive of the **amount of time** these activities actually took. So, time spent riding in the car seemed like it could go on forever; worse still, there was nothing to *do* to anchor himself in time. So, he gave himself some-thing to do that would make noise, have a sequence, and fill the endless gap he perceived. He would pinch his brother—something to do that was within reach and would create a sequential response; brother cries, mom yells, then she lectures, and the next thing you know, he's at the store and the ride is over. As Paul developed concepts of time, not only did he have a better concept of the length of the ride, he was also able to mentally place himself in *other* situations, engaging his mother about events at school that day, or asking what she needed from the store. Without a solid concept of time, events occurred sequentially, but seemingly without boundaries or connections to one another.

This could also help to explain why retaining information was so difficult for him. While his mother was working on letter-recognition with him, he would eventually begin to recall the information, but the next day that learning was gone and they had to start all over again. The learning activity was not separated in time from other activities and thus marked as significant by his brain. So, the events were not remembered, just as we don't remember the pedantic activities of getting dressed each morning.

After three months of treatment, Paul was independent with getting ready for school at his mother's request; meaning he understood that there was a finite amount of time before it was time to leave for school, and brushing teeth and dressing were the events that take about that much time.

Paul's time-awareness developed on both the micro and the macro level, concurrently. At the macro-level, a child needs an understanding of the timing of each day to construct the meaning found in planning for the school week, understanding the seasons and looking forward to events. This time-awareness development also happens across much shorter time intervals, and it is the understanding of the smaller intervals that allow communication and speech development, attention across the amount of time required to understand an idea (such as the sequence of a story), or the development of self-control to wait for something forthcoming.

It may seem that time-awareness is innate because no one "teaches" it to us. The brain is not born knowing time concepts; instead they are built on the foundation of auditory processing. One learns the meaning behind words by listening to others speak. One learns to attend to a story read to them because they want to know how it ends. One learns to wait because they have waited in small increments and those increments become longer as a person gathers more experiences. However, if a child does not possess the most elemental concept of time, as developed through awareness of rhythm and space between sounds, then all of these expected outcomes do not occur. Remember, we can only learn by connecting new information to that which we already know. A child without the beginning of time-concept development, as achieved through auditory processing, does not connect spoken sounds from others into meaningful words, does not develop the ability to listen to a story, and might not be able to accept waiting as a common occurrence in daily life.

The concepts outlined above and Paul's story require many leaps of faith that science has yet to fully articulate and justify. However, in framing the behaviors of children as a function of auditory skills and deficits, and addressing those skills and deficits directly, a child gathers the ability to construct higher level skills, like attention and learning, for themselves. The entire process is more organic and less frustrating for the child and the adults in their lives.

For those of you who caught the reference in the title of this chapter, HAL 9000 was the computer in Arthur C. Clarke's novel and movie *2001: A Space Odyssey*. If you'll remember, HAL began making decisions for the crew of the spaceship, because "his" judgment was better than the poor, flawed humans. It's a bit creepy when the astronaut issues a command to HAL and the computer responds calmly with, "I'm sorry, Dave, but I can't let you do that." I often think that might be what it is like for a child who *wants* to attend and learn, who *wants* to behave well and care for others. But their brain is making decisions without their permission, because of faulty processing. If, through appropriate therapy, we could return some of the control of a child's brain and body to them, then they would have the ability and the opportunity to learn, make good decisions and express who they are within.

5 The Ear Organizes the Brain and Body

Because the element of time is crucial in comprehending what sounds mean in a given situation, it is the foundation for our understanding of sequencing. It is the introduction of the concepts of **"before" and "after,"** before a child has even learned the words for those concepts. In the womb, sounds and the spaces between them lay the foundation for the most important sequence of action in a newborn's young life; the suck-swallow-breathe pattern that must be established for a newborn to time the rhythmic sequence of drawing milk from a nipple, swallowing it, and taking a pause to breathe. If this sequence does not develop appropriately, a newborn might have trouble staying latched to the nipple, swallowing safely, or sustaining the endurance required to complete a full intake of sustenance.

Interestingly, for children who were born prematurely, it has been found that listening to a piece of music with a tempo of 70 beats-per-minute helps to support longer, more effective feeding sessions. This is the average heart rate for a woman at rest. Is it possible that the maternal heart-rate in utero is setting the stage for a baby's understanding of rhythm, and after birth a baby applies this understanding to the very new task of eating? Again, our brains can only scaffold new learning on top of existing knowledge, so it would certainly make sense that the mother's heart rate might be the baby's best point of reference for how quickly to suck-swallow-breathe.

As a baby develops, the brain uses its established understanding of rhythm to place sounds into the correct sequence within a situation, helping to build their database files. The auditory circuits of the brain must sequence sounds correctly into words and songs

---

Suck-Swallow-Breathe and <u>Picky Eating</u>

The ability to effectively nurse after birth is directly related to an understanding of rhythm and sequencing. The suck-swallow-breathe pattern that allows a baby to alternate between oxygen consumption and food consumption is very rhythmic, and awareness of rhythm is established through hearing. Children who are older but have a history of poor latching and feeding may still be struggling with the oral motor skills and timing of how to chew, breathe, move food around their mouths and swallow. That's a lot to accomplish when you're not sure if you might choke or not be able to breathe when your body tells you to. And those difficulties can be further compounded by the lack of oral motor skills and sensory awareness that can happen when a child doesn't have an accurate feeling of where they are and how their body feels. These are factors to consider for children who have trouble eating or a history of food rejection.

---

for those sounds to have meaning. This unconscious sequencing is the beginning of our brain's understanding of sequencing at the conscious level as well. Sound helps us realize that one moment or event must precede another to make sense of our world. The ear helps the brain to sequence sounds, and eventually events, across time.

At the fastest levels of sequence processing, the brain reconstructs separate neural impulses into coherent words by placing the impulses into the correct sequence. As an example, if I say the word "pitch", my mouth produces three distinct sounds. The /p/ sound is generated at a primary frequency of about 1200 cycles per second (Hertz, or Hz). This frequency of soundwaves enters the ear and is changed to a single neural impulse and sent to the brain. The /i/ sound occurs at about 600 Hz; a second, separate neural impulse. Then the /ch/ sound, at 1500 Hz, creates a third neural impulse. The brain has to take these three distinct impulses and order them correctly to hear the word "pitch", before its meaning can be understood as a word. If the sequencing of those sounds is not correct or consistent, then perhaps one might hear the word "chip."

In addition, the brain must also sequence the word into the greater context of the situation or the sentence. The word "pitch" could mean a sound, or it could mean the act of throwing a ball. The word's placement in the scenario and within the sentence are all important sequencing factors that the brain learns to analyze to understand language. When a child learns language, they are also learning the fundamental principles of the sequencing of events, objects and patterns.

Some children with autism have difficulty with sequencing, being unable to connect one sound or sensation with another across a continuum of time. Many people with autism are "associational thinkers"; instead of an image or sound being related to the sound or image that came before or after, each sensation stimulates a memory of another, seemingly unrelated, image or idea. This may happen because their experience with sequencing and time as a function of hearing has been impaired. In his book *The Reason I Jump*, Naoki Higashida writes, "...I very quickly forget what it is I've just heard. Inside my head there really isn't such a big difference between what I was told just now, and what I heard a long, long time ago" (p.10). Temple Grandin also writes about her sequencing difficulties and her need to read aloud in her youth to keep the proper sequence of words and ideas (p.103).

When the brain can't sequence auditory information, it begins to have a difficult time deciding what information to attend, and what to "skip over." For example, when listening to a sentence such as, "I took the dog for a long walk today," one's brain naturally discards words like "the" and "a" so that the meaning of "long" (as opposed to short) and "today" (as opposed to last week), can be processed as relevant to the situation. The situation may be, "Has the dog had enough exercise lately?" When words congeal to form concepts that begin to answer implied or explicit questions, the processing of information can happen at higher cognitive levels, and not involve such specific, perceptual processing by the brain.

There is evidence that people with dyslexia and learning disabilities may have trouble forming these higher-level cognitive associations. For a long while after **dyslexia** was named as a condition, it was thought to develop from visual-perceptual deficits—that people with dyslexia have trouble reading because they are receiving faulty information from their eyes. Through further research, underlying auditory-perceptual (also called *psychoacoustic*) deficits were found to play a role in reading and learning difficulties. Tasks like isolating speech from background noise or pitch discrimination were thought to make reading difficult. From a more recent study, however, a new concept of dyslexia is evolving. In 2006, Ahissar et al. found that people with dyslexia and concurrent learning disabilities performed just as well as controls on tasks of sound comparison and frequency discrimination.

Where they struggled was in comparing repetitive sounds. In control groups (those without dyslexia), recognizing and retrieving cognitive representations of sound was easier in shorter bursts (in essence, the control group's brains recognized the sounds in shorter bursts more easily than in longer sequences) and they performed better on tests involving these skills. However, the dyslexic group did not benefit from shorter sets of information, and performed just as poorly on auditory recall on short sets of information as long ones. This poor performance in recognizing repeated speech sounds in short bursts correlated with poor scores in working memory and attentional tasks. The researchers concluded that both problems could be a result of an inability in the brains of dyslexics to form auditory "perceptual anchors." These perceptual anchors are the speech patterns that people without learning disabilities automatically recognize, because they are files in their database.

Could it be that impaired ability to sequence incoming speech sounds limits pattern recognition in speech? If the brain can't easily recognize and file patterns, it might be overtaxed in the areas of attention and processing. If it were possible to help a person's brain more easily establish sequential processing and pattern-recognition, then more attentional effort could be devoted to higher cognitive processes. In other words, if a dyslexic person's brain processed speech sequences and patterns more easily, could they focus on the *meaning* of what they hear and read, as opposed to the *perception* of what they hear and read?

In a young child's brain, processing of the sounds around them leads to the development of time concepts and sequencing abilities. Eventually children become adept enough in these abilities to begin to process speech. While speech is *unpredictable,* insofar as it expresses unique ideas from the mind of an individual, it is also fairly *predictable* within a language and culture. Certain groups speak with certain speeds and cadences, using similar words and grammar. As a child's brain begins to recognize the sequence and patterns common in everyone's speech, they begin to use those same patterns to communicate information within their own heads.

This wonderful development only happens if they begin to move the processing of sound to higher levels of cognitive processing. According to Schnupp, Nelken and King (2012), "the auditory system is thought to decipher speech sounds through a hierarchy of successive analyses, which operate on different timescales" (p.175). A *directive* is issued quickly: "Don't touch that!" which can be processed as lower brain centers as a warning to protect one's safety, a low-level brain function. An *idea* takes longer to communicate, and working memory must become involved: "A rabbit lives in a warren, which is a den underground where the rabbit's entire family lives together. It is protected from predators and weather because it is underground." Understanding this new learning involves the recall of complex ideas such as family, protection, and underground.

When the brain is "stuck" in lower levels of processing, such as attending to the actual sound of individual words, higher levels of cognitive processing aren't engaged. This limits a person's ability to form and access verbal memories. Many times, this lack of processing at higher brain levels results in **echolalia**, a condition in which a child will, seemingly endlessly, repeat a phrase that they have heard. This phrase may have a specific meaning for them because of its association with some non-sequential experience, or it may mean nothing at all. But it is essentially *not* communication, because the idea the words are meant to convey is not recognizable by most people.

So why do some children have difficulty forming these word-idea database files that allow for easy retrieval of ideas when they hear a word or want to communicate an idea? A look at the neural processing of sound within the brain reveals several places in which the train of information from the ear to the database may breakdown.

From Perception to Attention to Memory

Think back to the doorbell example from earlier in this book regarding how adults process the orienting response, but this time let's take a look at that scenario through the eyes of the child playing in the room. Let's say the child is 18 months old, and doesn't have a lot of experience hearing the doorbell. At the sound of the bell, the child will be alerted in an obvious way. They will stop what they are doing, hold still for a moment, and raise their eyes. The sound will be difficult to locate, and even if they are able to locate the source, it's the bell mounted to a wall somewhere, not the door. But they have perceived a change in their environment. If they have 18 months of dependably accurate auditory information up to this point and they are developing a dependable sound-vision database, their attention will continue to focus on this new information until the "what is that noise and what does it mean?" mystery is solved. Once (or perhaps twice) that Mom has gone to the door at the sound of the bell, memory, and therefore learning, will be achieved as the child correctly associates the sound with the meaning of someone being at the door. Bingo! Sound-database file created.

Closing this sound-vision loop is extremely important to new learning, and the paramount skill involved is **sound localization**. An accurate system for locating the source of sound is how babies and children develop their sound database. Not only must a child be able to locate a sound-source within their environment with specificity, they must also be able to access their sound-database easily and choose to attend to a stimulus long enough to form a memory. Referencing an accurate sound database is very helpful when children are choosing to attend to something visually.

The McGurk effect illustrates the strong brain connections made between the ear and the eye. This effect is the illusion that occurs when one hears a consonant-vowel combination, such as the sound "da", overlaid with the visual image of a person's mouth making the sound "la." Because of the strong sound-sight database most of us have established, the resulting sound perceived will be "la", even if the soundtrack played is clearly "da", which can be easily perceived if one closes their eyes to eliminate the conflicting visual input. These dominant visual images are created as sound database files for most people, so that we can "wade through" other's variable accents, variable emphases, and variable vocal tones as they are speaking our language. This helps the brain make sense of the different ways the same sentence can be said by someone from Boston, London or New Orleans. But it also illustrates the strength of the neural connections created by our eyes and ears as we make sense of the world through our sound database.

Learning which mouth shapes make which sounds is highly contingent on a very accurate sound localization ability. To create these sight-sound connections, a child must focus her eyes on an area of space that is about four square inches out of the full 360-degree surround. The brain locates a sound down to a very specific point through several neural mechanisms built on the natural characteristics of sound.

How do we know where a sound is coming from with so much specificity? It's a very complex process, but at the most rudimentary level, a sound generated on our right side will hit our right ear first, then our left. The time difference between the sound's reception in each ear can begin to tell us how far to the right or left that sound is. The brain can measure *very* small differences in the timing of sounds, down to below 700 microseconds (Schnupp et al, p. 143). This is the time difference between a sound from the right hitting a person's right ear, and then the left, if said person's head is pretty large. For a child's small head, the time gap between ears is even shorter. And if the sound is not coming directly from the right, but perhaps more toward the middle, the time gap will be even smaller. Sound localization is initiated by this time differential between sound hitting one ear, then the other. But, to get the muscles of the eye to focus on a specific point, more information from the sound must be processed. There are several specialized areas of the brain devoted to analyzing incoming sound for localization cues. The perception of the subtle difference of a sound's source from one side of our head to the other is the responsibility of our **lateral superior olive (LSO)**. The LSO is an olive-shaped (surprise!) node in the midbrain that analyzes differences between one ear and the other. Put simply, the LSO compares the information between ears and "chooses" which ear is likely closer to the sound based on whether the sound information is coming directly to the ear, or through or around the head, indicated by a difference in the level of sound volume. Once an ear has been chosen as the "listening ear", the brain sends inhibitory impulses to the opposite ear so that the brain does not get confused by the continuing conflicting information.

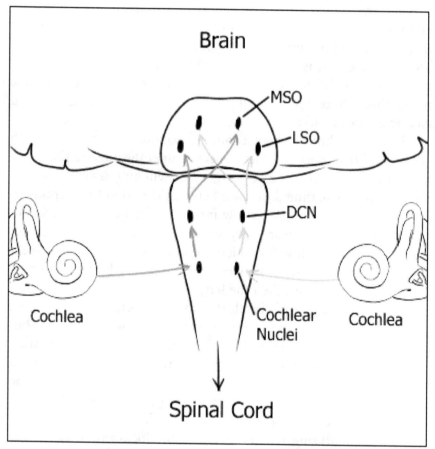

Fig. 5-1: Partial neural pathway for auditory input

Because low-frequency (lower-pitched) sound waves travel with greater energy, they propagate through the head and outer ear fairly well. This leaves very little difference between ears for the LSO to compare. However, there is a greater difference between ears when higher-frequency sound (like speech) is involved. This makes the LSO key in locating speech sources in our surround, because vocal noises are higher in pitch than background or "white" noise.

While the LSO is responsible for locating sound in the horizontal plane, sound comes from above and below head-level as well. The dorsal cochlear nucleus (DCN) is the brain structure that listens to the entire auditory surround, including the variations in a particular sound, listening for the most direct route of the sound from its source to the ear. In an enclosed or crowded space, a sound will reflect off objects and walls as it emanates from the source. These reflections distort and throw the sound waves out of rhythm. But there is one pathway from the sound source to the ear that is most distinct. The DCN's role is to locate this "cleanest" sound from the full spectrum of sound the ear receives. This includes recognizing when a sound source is located behind us, as the sound has to travel through and around the outer ear, known as the pinna. This helps the brain determine not only the sound's source around our head in the horizontal plane, in front or behind; but also the vertical, below or above.

In the brainstem, which evolved from the brains of rather skittish reptiles as the theory goes, a low-frequency sound may indicate as much of a threat as a high-frequency sound, and therefore must be located with some accuracy as well. The brain accomplishes this through another method of ear-comparison, the intra-aural time difference. To understand intra-aural time differences, it helps to visualize sounds as waves, which have crests a set distance apart.

When a sound comes from the left, the crest of the sound wave will hit the left ear drum a miniscule fraction of a second before the crest hits the right ear drum. The brain measures this time difference as a fraction of the time between wave-crests. Because the crests of

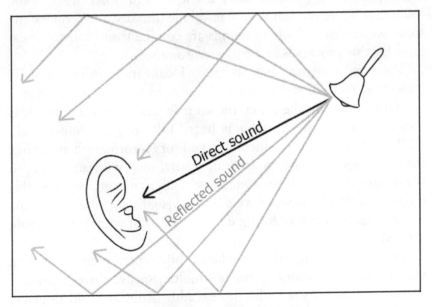

Fig. 5-2: Direct vs. reflected sound.

low-frequency sounds are further apart, the brain has a longer amount of time to "measure" between ears to guess how far and from where a sound might be emanating. Therefore, intra-aural time differences are more accurate when locating low-frequency sound sources, and this task falls mainly to brain structure known as the **medial superior olive (MSO)**.

Closing the Loop

While there are other brain structures involved, most elementally, the LSO, DCN and MSO work simultaneously to accomplish the complex task of locating the source of sound, no matter the position or frequency. Our brains can very accurately match the visual and auditory source of a sound; closing the auditory-visual loop and creating a file of information in our database. Because the ears and brain can locate almost any sound within the environment, the information is paired with ocular-motor muscles and visual input to create an accurate map of our surroundings.

As mentioned previously, sound processing in the brain runs along multiple neural tracks simultaneously. Some tracks are designed to analyze the temporal (timing and duration) aspects of sound and some process spectral (tone and pitch) information. These processing patterns make branches into other areas of the brain that figure out our spatial envelope (the size and scope of the space we are in) and where sounds are coming from. The technical term for this process is *auditory scene analysis*.

There is evidence that, because localization information is important to both the visual and auditory systems in creating a spatial map within the brain, the same location information file is created whether the stimulus is heard OR seen (Schnupp et al., p.207). Thus, we can use incoming auditory information about our surroundings to create an accurate spatial map without having to constantly observe our environment visually. You can see where this might come in handy when we'd like to visually concentrate on one point in space, without losing our awareness of what is happening around us.

Until about the age of four, when a child is presented with both a visual and an auditory stimulus simultaneously, their brain will register the auditory stimulus more readily (Robinson and Sloutsky, 2007). But perhaps a child is building an important sound-vision connection, such as learning tone of voice and its connection to facial expression. In these cases, a child would want to intentionally keep their visual focus on a person and not have to take their eyes away to monitor their environment. If they can depend on their ears to do the monitoring for them, then they can maintain their gaze and make visual learning connections more easily.

Other than when a child is focused on objects and events to form solid sound-sight connections, their eyes are almost never still. Their eyes are moving from near to far focus quite often. Typically, a child's eyes are not physiologically ready to near-focus for long periods until they are at least six or seven years old. This make sense developmentally, as a child should be continuing to explore their larger world physically, when they are meant to be developing and refining large muscle groups for overall body coordination. To maximize the time spent in this important development, they shouldn't be sitting for long periods to read or (UGH!) play on a screen, such as an iPad. **Long-period screen time** is developmentally detrimental; it has been shown to limit speech development, shorten attention span, and contribute to ADHD (Weiss et al., 2011). In addition, it creates a situation in which a child's eyes are stationary for long periods. But hearing one's environment and responding with vision and eye movement is crucial to developing depth-perception, ocular-motor control and head-neck-body control. Activities that don't complete the loop of the orienting response to hear and react with the body and eyes don't reinforce proper development.

There is evidence that children creating these sound/vision information files *must* look to the source of the sound to "close the loop"—for their brain to solidify the connection between sound and location. As early as 1980, scientists had established that children must look to the source of the sound to create a frame of reference for new learning about their environment, but a 1992 study at the University of Toledo found that "the precision of auditory localization may depend on the precision required of the resulting behavior" (Heffner and Heffner, p. 225) This means that the human brain best localizes sound when interaction with the environment is called for; be it looking for the source of the sound, touching objects from which sound reflects, or intercepting moving sources of sound (such as avoiding cars while crossing the street).

Neurological connections between hearing and looking also involve moving. A baby's muscle-control development begins at the top and moves downward. As a newborn lies on the floor or is held supported upright, they turn their head in response to sound, thus learning about control of the neck muscles. As they begin to work against gravity, on their tummies and eventually in sitting, it is this listening-looking loop that encourages movement around their center, both at the neck and torso level. This helps develop seated balance, fine muscle control and stability in various positions. All of these are necessary to develop even more discrete muscle movements, such those involved in holding a crayon, buttoning or brushing one's teeth.

When this listening-looking loop breaks down, it can negatively impact the way a child's eyes move. Sometimes the visual difficulty a child is having is subtle, such as slow progress with reading or being academically delayed. Perhaps a child has a more obvious difficulty, like strabismus (congenitally crossed-eyes) or amblyopia (lazy eye). I was very surprised to find that, when I used spatially-recorded sound with children with Down Syndrome who also had **strabismus**, their eyes became better aligned with each other. In one case, the young man had already had three surgeries to help align his eyes, with little success, but his gaze improved markedly through auditory therapy.

Babies in Buckets

Looking at how motor skills develop from an auditory perspective might make us rethink modern child-rearing. Consider the proliferation of plastic baby carriers in the last 20 to 30 years. Therapy professionals sometimes refer to this phenomenon as "babies in buckets." Babies are often placed in the carrier at home, placed in the car, lifted from the car and placed in a holder in a store or restaurant, then placed back in the car. For these hours, baby had little to no opportunity to engage the muscles of his core and neck to take in his environment. Auditory cues *should* initiate very frequent repetitions of head turning and eye coordination to locate the source of the sound, closing the listening-moving-looking loop of exploration that spurs physical development in infants.

Because the matching of visual and auditory input is dependent on making neural connections, the steps of this sensory-match ballet can be "tricked" and re-wired incorrectly. Sound sources can be "mis-located" if a sound is presented with a visual stimulus that is slightly off-target (Bertelson and Radeau, 1981). This trickery and its ensuing neural complications was studied in ferrets, in which the descending neural pathways were destroyed, and the result was impaired learning (Bajo et al., 2010). Think about that for a second. The information coming in to the ferrets' ears was not altered, but their neurological response to be able to concentrate on important information *was* impaired, and their learning of new information was impacted. What could that mean for children with learning problems? It is not the *input* that is creating difficulties, but the internal control mechanisms that allow for increased attention to important information. For me, this points directly to the reason for my frustration in working on attention and learning difficulties from a cognitive perspective. A child must have tremendous neurological control to *make* themselves concentrate against a potentially disrupted listening-looking-learning loop. If we could correct the loop for them through auditory therapy, wouldn't that be kinder?

Batman: Being Your Own Superhero

If child is hesitant to climb onto play equipment, or becomes anxious or upset whenever their feet are off the ground, such as when someone they don't emotionally trust lifts them up, the clinical term for this is **gravitational insecurity**. A child with gravitational insecurity might miss out on the developmental opportunities that children naturally take advantage of, like sliding and swinging at the playground or balancing while walking on a curb or retaining wall. Traditionally, the therapy community addressed this problem as a vestibular or balance issue, which seems to make sense initially. It appears that the gravitationally insecure child knows his balance is precarious and is afraid to challenge it because the likelihood of falling is high.

As explored briefly earlier, sound reflecting back to the ear is our initial exposure to the concept of distance, and our *visual* depth perception is built on top of that experience. I believe that, children in my clinic with visual depth-perception or visual-tracking problems (often manifested as reading difficulties), are actually having trouble locating distances *auditorily*.

However, in my experience, the anxiety or fear that results from climbing even a few inches off the ground is may be auditory in nature. The child is anxious because he doesn't inherently know how far away the ground is once his feet have left it. He might cognitively know he can step off the platform, but he doesn't have an instinctive understanding of whether he is six inches from the ground, or twelve inches from the ground. If he's only three feet tall, that's a big difference. The anxiety is related to a lack of auditory information about distance, not fear of losing his balance. I came to this conclusion after treating many gravitationally insecure children using sound for other reasons, only to see their insecurity surprisingly resolve itself.

Again, Naoki Higashida provides an insight into what might be an auditory processing deficit by explaining how his world with autism looks to him. Higashida suggests that a person with autism might perform the frequent action of "borrowing" someone else's hand to indicate or reach for an object because the person with autism doesn't know how far to extend their own hand to reach the desired object. He says, "[People with autism] have problems perceiving and gauging distances" (p.52).

The use of direct and indirect sound helps develop our depth perception, but it is also part of **echolocation,** which many animals such as bats and owls use to augment poor eyesight or to hunt at night. For both animals and humans, our brains paint a three-dimensional model of the space we are in, based on how sound bounces back to us. Our hearing is the first source of information regarding how far away an object or surface might be. As we build a sound-vision database, hearing becomes the secondary "fact-checker" for what we see with our eyes. When this database is unreliable for a child; and the resulting behaviors can appear to be fear of movement, anxiety, lack of attention and clumsiness. I often see children who are clumsy, bumping into objects like doorways and banging their head on objects; perhaps because they can't "hear" where the doorframe or objects are.

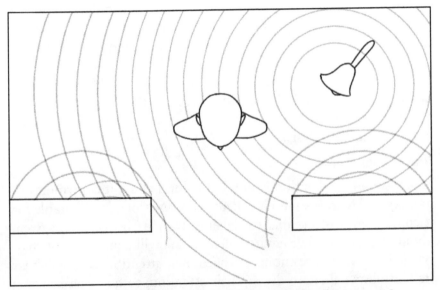

Fig. 5-3: "Hearing" an approaching doorway through reflected sound.

Imagine you are entering a very dark, unfamiliar room. You might subconsciously already know the approximate size of the room, whether it has carpet, or a high ceiling, and whether anyone else might be in it. If there is sufficient light, you can confirm all these qualities with your eyes. But what if you did not have sight? There is a man by the name of Dan Kish, who is blind but has a very well-developed sense of echolocation. He wows people by riding his bike through city streets, navigating by the sounds that bounce back to him from an audible clicking sound he makes. You can see a video of this on YouTube. He also has a Ted Talk that is pretty cool.

You might also notice that Dan Kish does not move his head side-to-side as many blind people do in the absence of a visual anchor (think Ray Charles or Stevie Wonder). He has an auditory anchor for the muscles of his head and neck. He moves fluidly and confidently through space. For the children in my clinic, their inability to move fluidly through their environment, rotate around their core, or climb onto surfaces above the ground with confidence can be traced back to poor spatial auditory processing through echolocation (along with perhaps inaccurate vestibular processing, which we will focus on in a later chapter).

Humans use echolocation, just like bats and dolphins, but it happens at a mostly subconscious level. It's possible that, before the advent of artificial light, humans were more in-tune with their skills of echolocation, but because our sight is almost always available, we have learned to depend more on our eyes. However, the *development* of visual observation skills and the ability to monitor the environment for safety are still built on a foundation of accurate auditory scene analysis.

Pretty Good Guesses

When sound localization is unreliable for a child, it contributes to anxiety and fear. If sound localization is functional and reliable for a child, they will be able to develop their early warning system about changes in their environment. They will come to trust that, when a sound is close enough to need their attention, they will hear it. This allows them to divide their attention; to focus on learning new skills and taking in new information. Remember that the Orienting Response is always trying to answer the question, "Is this safe?" If a child cannot answer that using their auditory system, they must use their conscious brain, their vision and/or proprioception. That greatly limits the amount of available attention left for them to learn to say "milk" or tie their shoes. And it also means a constant vigilance regarding their environment that can be distracting and anxiety-producing.

I know I'm dealing with a child whose sound-localization is on the blink when they repeatedly ask, "What's that noise?" Most of the time the noise to which they are referring is not unusual or not a threat, it may just be a child playing in another room. But their brain isn't able to filter noises accurately, their early-warning system doesn't work, and they must bring each noise to the level of consciousness to be analyzed. It's no wonder that these children come to me with anxiety, communication or learning difficulties. Their auditory sense is taking up too much of their working brain energy for them to have attention left over for learning or to be able to disengage and relax.

For the scientists among you, the leap between the concrete research on very discrete facets of the listening process, and the larger idea that these systems can breakdown and result in certain behaviors may be difficult to make. Additionally, there is no conclusive proof that the types of auditory therapy available actually work to correct the auditory-processing difficulties a child may be having. However, clinically, when I have used sound to address difficulties a child is having, I often find that, not only do the specific deficits we are addressing improve, but the child's comfort within the world, fluidity of movement and general level of happiness appear to improve. When I have addressed depth perception and sound localization through auditory therapy, I have observed increases in reading skills, improved self-care, such as dressing independently, or greater emotional expression range; even if these are skills we have not yet addressed through other methods. These are the times when academic journals are not my teachers, but children and families are. The following two children and their families were wonderful teachers.

Lucy

Lucy, almost four years old, had striking large brown eyes and a kind heart. Her mother was concerned about her limited vocabulary, rote social interactions, and articulation problems. As an infant, she had multiple ear infections and special tubes were placed in her eardrums when she was two. Her most persistent behavior during our initial time together, however, was a continual concern for where her mother was. Even if she was in the room with us, Lucy would **anxiously** ask, "Where's Mommy?" and look around for her every minute or two, causing an evident interruption to Lucy's train of thought and participation.

During the evaluation, I noticed that Lucy was gravitationally insecure and had poor ocular-motor skills. This, combined with her verbal articulation delays and limited vocabulary indicated that her auditory system was not providing accurate information. Lucy's therapeutic course began with nature-based sounds through headphones to help her practice echolocation, so that the skill would become more accurate when the headphones were off. Thus, she could more accurately move her eyes to points in space and be more consistent in perceiving depth. As she developed a better understanding of what was around her, she depended less on her mother to act as her early-warning system. Her focus on where her mom was decreased and she was able to participate in games that involved communication and sequences. As her fear diminished, we were able to move more in therapy and her tolerance to movement increased. By two months of treatment, she was able to come up with new motor plans based on changing information, her speech was clearer and she was less anxious. Just before discontinuing therapy at 3 months, Lucy's mom reported that they had attended a festival and Lucy needed to be monitored because it was likely she might wander away to go see something new. This independent exploration was very new and her mother was happy to see her daughter experiencing new environments without fear.

Brian

Brian had already been through kindergarten once and was on his second time through. He still struggled with learning the material, and his mother was frustrated by his inability to retain any information from day-to-day. He didn't recognize letters of the alphabet beyond the letter "C." He was diagnosed with ADHD (inattentive type) after many years of behavioral and social difficulties. His behavior had improved throughout the school year last year, but he continued to have trouble pronouncing many words, needed constant company and attention, and was very anxious about things that were unlikely to happen. Before bed some nights, he would ask his mother not to jump out the window during the night, and no amount of rational discussion could ease his **anxiety**. In short, he was wearing his mother out.

During our evaluation, I noticed that he was very easily visually distracted, leading me to conclude that the early-warning system of his hearing wasn't reliable. He had a poor awareness of time, becoming engrossed in sensations and losing a sense of what he was supposed to be doing. His ocular-motor skills were limited, and he struggled to hold his head still while moving his eyes around, indicating poor awareness of the muscles of his midline.

After a month of treatment, his ocular-motor skills improved, but he was having to contract *all* the muscles of his neck to stabilize his head, and that looked very uncomfortable. He was also still unable to judge distances well, stepping off a climbing wall when he was too far from the ground to be safe. To address these problems, we added spatially-enhanced soundscapes to his auditory therapy. The next month, his head movement was more stable, and he was identifying 90% of letters, which is acceptable for his age, and his pronunciation errors stopped altogether. By the end of therapy, Brian had ocular-motor skills sufficient to play catch effectively and his mother was thrilled that he also not only wanted to play basketball on a team, but that he was just as coordinated as the other children.

In both of these cases, the child's mother had previously sought out other therapies or tutoring, and nothing else about their routine had changed over the two to three months of therapy. But both children gained skills that were global and self-reinforcing in nature. Because Lucy was better able to judge distances, she moved more fluidly around her environment and was less anxious, thus creating more opportunities for more movement. Because Brian could move his eyes more easily to visual targets, he was able to create more accurate sound-letter database files and increase his learning, which increased his feelings of efficacy and his belief that he could learn more. For both children, their increased skill at monitoring their environment auditorily meant decreased anxiety and greater voluntary attention. While the science may not have caught up with what I have observed in the clinic, I consider children like Lucy and Brian to be evidence enough to attempt similar therapy with children who are having similar struggles.

A consistently functional auditory system is essential to normal brain development and behavior, but there is another piece of the puzzle of function that we have yet to explore. One half of the brain's GPS system, the auditory sense, gives the brain a mental map of the surrounding area and what is important in it. The vestibular system is the other half of the GPS system. It creates the brain's "You Are Here" dot on the map, and it has a significant influence on emotion, behavior, communication and movement. We've put the cart before the horse a bit here by investigating the role of the auditory system in brain and body development, but we had to start somewhere. In the ensuing chapters, let's turn our attention to the horse, the vestibular system.

6 Introducing the Vestibular System

"When something goes wrong in the neural functions that relate us to gravity, most people attribute the resulting problem to some other cause."
— Jean Ayres, the founder of Sensory Integration Therapy, in *Sensory Integration and the Child*

As an experiment, move to exit the room you're in and stop directly on the threshold of the doorway. As you do this, think about the planning involved. Locating the doorway (which involves being aware of your surround and having appropriate ocular-motor skills), estimating the steps remaining to get to the threshold (which can be done visually, based on the speed with which the doorway seems to be approaching), and knowing when you need to slow down to achieve stillness just when you want to (which can be sensed proprioceptively—using your muscles and joints). Now, as you stop, pay attention to the muscles involved in halting your forward momentum, and all the associated muscles that have to contract to keep from using *too much* force to stop, and actually falling backward. These split-second reactions can only be processed and executed accurately by using vestibular information (coming from the vestibulae of the inner ears). In fact, it is a unique feature within the body that the vestibular system has such a quick response time. The neurons that come from the vestibular centers in the brain are noticeably faster at transmitting their information than other sensorimotor neurons in the body.

The other two methods of orientation in space, vision and proprioception, require more cognitive processing and depend on potentially unreliable information. The visual method of orientation could break down due to movement occurring beyond the doorway, or if it is limited by low lighting. The proprioceptive system can be

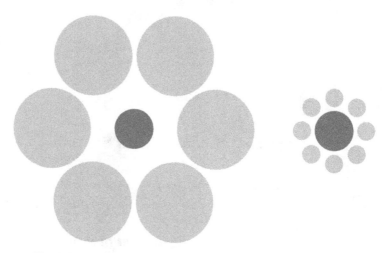

Fig. 6-1: The circles in the center really are the same size.

thrown off by a change in walking surface, such as hard floor to carpeting, or a floor that leads to a ramp. But the vestibular system can react with accurate information for the body to use quickly and reliably, because of its more direct connections between the brain and the skeletal muscles.

Using other methods of situational awareness are often not as accurate. You can see this for yourself when you look at an optical illusion like the one above, in which both central circles are the same size. Really. If you had to depend solely on what you see to navigate the world, your eyes wouldn't always be a dependable source of information.

Here is another experiment to try. Close your eyes and, keeping your elbows straight, try to bring your index fingers to one another in front of you. This is a completely proprioceptive maneuver; you can't use your vision to adjust the course of your arms as they move. In theory, you should already know where both fingers are in space, because they are both sending you proprioceptive information. But most people cannot do this because the proprioceptive system doesn't provide that kind of precision. Another version of this task is to try to touch your elbow with you opposite index finger without looking.

For children who might not be receiving or processing vestibular information effectively, the unreliability of proprioceptive and visual information may help to explain why they are clumsy, use too much force for tasks, struggle with either gross or fine motor tasks (or sometimes both), and in general don't move as smoothly as they should. It is possible that, instead of augmenting accurate information from their vestibular system, the visual and proprioceptive systems are providing all the information they use to navigate the world.

The Vestibular System Already Has Street Cred

One of the unique contributions of Sensory Integration Theory was its emphasis on the vestibular system. By bringing attention to this unexplored sensory system, therapists, educators and parents could now consider sensory input beyond the "five senses" taught in school. Vestibular input affects a child's ability to learn, to remain calm, to participate safely in social situations, and myriad other daily activities. Because we all depend upon an accurate vestibular system to function, therapists began applying Sensory Integration treatment *beyond* children with learning disabilities—to children with autism, ADHD, and other diagnoses.

The vestibular system is a complicated sensory system that we typically don't learn much about in school. It can be challenging for some people to understand just how much this system does for us all day, every day, because for most of us this system functions well. When the vestibular system is functioning well enough to keep us engaged appropriately in our daily life, we aren't *supposed* to notice it. It is like the operating system of a computer. It's in the background, making sure our keystrokes and mouse-clicks get directed to the proper circuit. We only interact with the interface of the computer—our bodies, our hands, our eyes, our voice—trying to accomplish our goals using our bodies as a tool to express our will. We can't sense the actions of our vestibular system in the background, coordinating the interactions of our bodies with the world; much as we don't see the actions of our computer's operating systems.

However, there are times when, even for neurotypical people, the vestibular system *does* malfunction. Those moments can help us conceive of what daily life might be like for a child with difficulties. If you develop an ear infection, or vertigo, or Meniere's disease, the resulting dizziness will certainly get your attention. Even the temporary sensation of being drunk, which affects your vestibular system, can throw off your movement, coordination and timing, making it hard to trust your body to coordinate interactions with your environment. Remember that *you* are noticing these sensory systems "acting funny" because you can compare the sensations to how you feel when everything is working well. Your child may have never been able to use his vestibular system to provide accurate information.

Because we seldom notice our functional vestibular system, it is helpful to explore examples of how vestibular function contributes to our daily activities. Then, we can understand how disruption of vestibular input might affect children. First, a working knowledge of this system's anatomy and physiology is necessary. Keep in mind that the auditory and vestibular systems are not truly separate. For the purposes of discussion, I am dividing the vestibular from the auditory, but from an anatomical and physiological perspective the vestibular and auditory system are so closely linked as to be considered the same system. They are both housed in the same place, deep within the skull, in our inner ear, surrounded by the hardest bone in our body, the temporal bone. We have both vestibular and auditory end organs (receptors) on each side of our head. Both the auditory and vestibular receptors serve the same function: to sense movement.

The auditory end organ, the cochlea, senses fine movements in the air (sound waves) which our brains translate through neural impulses as sound. The vestibular end organ has specially shaped fluid-filled tubes and pouches that sense larger movements of our head through space. These movements can occur in several planes; around our core (rotation), vertically and horizontally. The cross-over point between the auditory and vestibular systems is vibration, which is both low frequency sound and high frequency movement that can be both heard and felt. Recall the sensation of sitting in traffic when a car drives up behind you with the stereo loud and the bass turned up. Don't you hear it AND feel it in your seat? Can't you see the rearview mirror vibrating to the beat?

To keep things concise, we will treat these systems as separate from one another. But it is good to keep in mind how interconnected they are; to better understand why taking your child through a vestibular program can increase their communication ability, or how an auditory program can improve coordination and posture.

The Anatomy of the Vestibular System

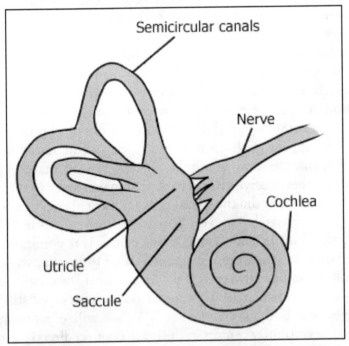

Semicircular canals

Nerve

Cochlea

Utricle

Saccule

Fig. 6-2: Anatomy of the Vestibular System in the Inner Ear

The vestibular system (Fig. 6-2) is composed of the saccule, utricle and semicircular canals. The utricle and saccule are designed to sense movement or stillness in the vertical and horizontal planes, such as when we are in car that takes off from a stop or in an elevator that begins to move vertically. The semicircular canals are designed to sense rotary acceleration, such as turning our head or tilting it down or up. The sensors in the semicircular canals sense any change in rate of movement over two revolutions per second (Clark, 2009). As an experiment, put this book down, stand up and spin around fast enough to make yourself dizzy. The dizziness doesn't really come from the act of spinning, but from the change in inertia created by starting and stopping spinning. That change in velocity, acceleration or deceleration, is pretty fast.

Once you've recovered from your dizziness, just once, turn your head to look directly to the right, as if someone has just called your name from the right. That movement is just as fast, if not more so;

it's just much shorter in duration. So, even though that head-turning movement was only about ⅕ to ¼ of a full rotation, your semicircular canals sensed the movement accurately. Your brain needs information about this movement—when it is happening and how large or small it is—so it can coordinate all the resulting muscles and sensations. This information helps to keep your eyes stable in your head, to know that any source of noise in the environment will also "move" around you as your ears rotate with your head, and to prepare the muscles in your neck and torso to accept the accompanying shift in the weight of your body.

All this happens fairly effortlessly, as long as the senses of your ears, eyes, muscles and vestibular system can all match up the information they receive into a puzzle that makes sense to the brain. Now, if you actually did the spinning experiment above, your senses started to "mismatch" as you got dizzy from spinning. This is because the fluid in your semicircular canals was coming to rest (telling you that you were not moving), due to inertia, while you were still spinning. However, your visual world was still on the move—sensory mismatch! Your vestibular system says "still" and your eyes and body say "moving." As we will explore in this chapter, the vestibular centers in the brain connect directly with the vagus nerve, which senses and controls much of the action in our stomach and intestines. This is why the sensory mismatch of getting dizzy can often result in nausea and vomiting. Perhaps it is also the reason we tend to describe vestibular sensations in terms of our stomach, as in "my stomach was in my throat" or "my stomach dropped."

While the semicircular canals provide feedback about rotational head movement, the utricle and saccule are constantly giving your brain feedback about the head's position in space to coordinate with vision, hearing and muscle sensations. Vestibular sensation is meant to "fact check" the accuracy of those other inputs. That's the job of the vestibular system. It gives your body a point of reference in space that is independent of any input other than gravity and movement. When sensations from your vestibular fact-checker don't make a coherent picture with your visual, proprioceptive, or auditory perception, the result can be anxiety, hyperarousal and/or physiological rejection, such as vomiting. Car sickness is a common example of this. Your utricle, which senses movement in the horizontal plane, is telling you that you are still. This information doesn't match the visual movement flashing by the car window. The utricle is sensing that you are stationary because of the inertia of your body traveling in the car, but your eyes are telling you, "We're moving! Fast!" That's a mismatch. Often in this situation, when a person moves to the front seat the sensation of carsickness subsides. In the front seat, the eyes can focus into the distance, which doesn't appear to be moving as quickly and is more visually stable.

For children who have a persistently dysfunctional vestibular system, the result is not usually vomiting or nausea, although sometimes these children can be more prone to those afflictions. More common behaviors are anxiety and emotional reactivity. Consider this example: you are pulling into a parking space at the grocery store. Unbeknownst to you, the driver of the car in the next parking space decides to pull his car out simultaneously with your car stopping. No doubt the sensory mismatch of feeling you are stopping, concurrent with the unexpected visual movement of the other car gives you a moment of slight panic and you might stomp down on the brake pedal. For some children, this low-level chronic anxiety or upset could be an all-day-long occurrence, as they are never 100% sure of their position in space, giving them regular sensory mismatches. Because most children are just learning to control and express their emotions, a child whose physical world that doesn't always feel stable might always be one slight, unexpected sensation away from a tantrum.

Little movements make a big difference

There are two important concepts to keep in mind when considering the influence of the vestibular system. First, it is extremely sensitive. The cochlea, the organ with which we hear, is designed to pick up air wave compressions that we cannot see nor feel on our skin. The sensors within the vestibulum are also sensitive to the slightest movement. Second, there are many projections from the vestibular system to different areas of the brain. It has a role in body position, motor coordination, spatial orientation, sleep, and ocular-motor (eye muscle) control. But its most important function is simply to tell us that we are safe in regard to movement; that we are not moving when we expect not to be moving and that we *are* moving when that is what is expected. In this way, it contributes to our sense of security and effectiveness, our feelings of control and ability to react easily to anything that might happen.

The vestibular system develops in the womb and is 100% functional (along with the auditory system) when a child is born, assuming the child is born after 24 weeks gestation. In utero, suspended in amniotic fluid, the baby feels the acceleration and deceleration of mom's movement, as well as his or her self-generated movements. This is the baby's first opportunity to make a sensory match between an externally-created sensation and the internal sense of position in space. Experiencing movement and gravity during the prenatal period allows a newborn to arrive in the outside world with already-established expectations about how gravity and acceleration affect their bodies. An exceptionally cool study conducted by Ronca et al. in 2008 studied pregnant rats who experienced gravity-free space flight, who then gave birth to vestbularly-impaired pups, leading researchers to conclude that prenatal movement experiences "shape prenatal organization and function within the mammalian vestibular system" (p.224). What might the implications be of this idea for mothers who are on bedrest for extended periods of time during pregnancy? Or those fetuses exposed to toxic substances during this formative period? Or children born very prematurely?

After birth, gravity becomes a force to be reckoned with, literally. Initially, a baby is most typically in a horizontal position, lying on a surface, and has the opportunity to feel the weight of their limbs and learn which muscles to contract and with how much force to control and stabilize them. This process is helped along by infant reflexes, such as the stepping reflex. This reflex causes a newborn baby to actively extend his leg when a surface comes into contact with the bottom of his foot. These automatic actions allow a baby to develop a sense of muscle strength and excursion. Until muscular control develops sufficiently, we swaddle newborns; if they want to rest, we have to give them some external feedback to keep those little limbs in check. As loved ones hold the baby in a supported upright position, the wee one learns which muscles support their head in upright. The brain compares this muscular feedback to the feeling of lifting their (seemingly much heavier) head when they are lying down. It certainly takes a lot more muscle contraction to lift the head from a lying position, and so they learn about center of gravity, lever-arm length, and the resulting need for force. With repeated practice, muscles strengthen and motor control increases.

This process of learning how to move against gravity with the appropriate force continues in little increments throughout childhood, even as children become old enough to sit in a chair, balance on curbs and retaining walls, and coordinate body and eye movements for ball sports. These millions of learning moments are based on accurate and consistent feedback from the vestibular system. If it is impaired, then the resulting data are not accurate, the correct neural pathways are not strengthened, and the child does not have an effective, or possibly even a successful, interaction with the world around them.

Just like auditory input, vestibular input gets distributed throughout the brain along multiple tracts simultaneously. Some connections may be easy to understand, such as the connections to eye and skeletal muscles. Other connections may be less intuitive, but may help explain the vestibular-systems influence on behaviors such as sleep, emotional stability, and memory formation.

The vestibular system provides "a unique and complete description of head motion and orientation in three dimensions," state Day and Fitzpatrick in their 2005 summation of the function of the vestibular system for the journal *Current Biology* (p.585), by providing information regarding:

- "Self" versus "non-self" motion (are we moving, or are things moving around us?)

- Spatial orientation

- Navigation

- Voluntary movement

- Ocular-motor (eye-movement) control.

The brain coordinates incoming sensations from all the sensory systems, based on vestibular input, to create a cohesive picture of where we are and where we are going. It is possible that, like auditory sensations, vestibular sensations create database files matched with

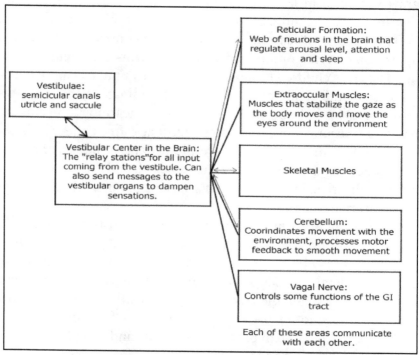

Fig. 6-3: The Neural connections of the Vestibular System

situations and other forms of sensory input. For example, there are separate neural patterns in the brain for head-direction and spatial orientation when travelling. Having two distinct neural pathways for the same situation makes sense if you consider an example. Imagine you have your head turned to speak to a friend with whom you are chatting while walking to get coffee. You are still effortlessly able to self-navigate to the coffee shop, even though your head is not turned in the direction you are travelling. This is because information from your semi-circular canals, which sense rotation of the head, converges with saccule-based information, regarding forward motion, creating a cohesive picture of "navigation to coffee shop" in your brain. If information about the direction of your head (and therefore your inner ear) was not also superimposed on information about your body's movement through space, you'd have a hard time getting to the coffee shop without keeping your head facing forward.

The chart on the previous page (Fig. 6-3) illustrates the many projections the vestibular system has with different structures of the brain and body. Keep in mind that these structures also communicate directly with each other, using the information provided by the vestibulae. Neural impulses from the vestibular nuclei (which receives the transmissions from the vestibular end organs) create a diffuse network of impulses throughout the brain simultaneously. This may explain why the vestibular system can influence functions and behaviors seemingly unrelated to balance and coordination.

Unfortunately, we can't flip open little heads to see exactly where the wires are routed and which ones are disconnected or misconnected. We can't take pliers and reconnect erroneous neural connections. One of the few ways we have to understand a child's vestibular function is to look at their resulting behaviors and preferences and make an educated guess. Sometimes, specific behaviors are a result of faulty information about security regarding movement and gravity. We can be more confident about our educated guesses when specific behaviors are positively affected by therapeutic movement. Such behaviors will be discussed in specific in subsequent chapters.

What Can Go Wrong?

What happens during development to create the neurological quirks that make it difficult for a child to use their vestibular system properly? Premature birth, chronic ear infections, chronic allergies, fetal substance exposure, autism, and ADHD are common in the medical histories of my clients. Any of these issues, or some other cause, can create a situation in which a child might have suppressed or inconsistent vestibular sensation. If information coming from the vestibular system isn't intense enough or isn't consistent, neural pruning may occur, weakening links between the vestibular centers and skeletal and/or ocular motor muscles. In a situation like this, the brain may begin to rely on visual and proprioceptive input as more reliable.

In early childhood, neural connections are formed and pruned rapidly, and connections continue to be made and destroyed by the body throughout our life, in a process known as **neural plasticity**. This is essentially what happens neurologically any time we learn something new. As we repeatedly practice what we learn, neural connections strengthen. Conversely, neural connections we *don't* use become weaker and may disappear completely. Donald Hebb, a

---

What We *Can* Measure

Because of the vestibular system's connection to the reticular formation and the vagal nerve, several research studies on children with sensory processing disorder (SPD) have focused on increased sweat production, increased salivary cortisol (a stress hormone that helps determine continuing stress after the cessation of a stressful stimulus) and heart rate variability. The idea behind this research is that children with SPD are always at a heightened state of arousal because their sensory systems don't provide input that their brain can trust, creating uncertainty and anxiety about the world. Indeed, researchers have found that difficulties in the inner ear, particularly the vestibular system, can create changes in the brain related to hyperactive and/or anxious behavior.

---

psychologist, famously said, "Neurons that fire together, wire together."

The difficulty that develops from a switch of information sources, from the vestibular system to the visual or proprioceptive system, is that the child loses the "fact-checker" verification that the vestibular system provides. The brain's decisions become based on information from senses that are not as quickly adaptable to change and are dependent on the outside world, which can be unreliable (as discussed at the beginning if this chapter). Our visual world can move, surfaces underneath us can change, both of which alter our perception. Depending only on information the brain cannot fact check means that a child will want that information to always be available. For example, some children cannot stand to get new shoes, or insist on being barefoot even when it's not safe, because they need the most reliable proprioceptive or tactile input to their feet to feel grounded and stable. These children are very dependent on their proprioceptive and tactile systems to engage with their environment, and this makes them less adaptable when the requirements of their environment change; such when Dad needs them to wear shoes to keep their feet off hot pavement.

Not only is the vestibular system the fact-checker for physical experiences we are having, it also helps us predict what *will* happen in the physical world. In their 2005 summary of the functions of the vestibular system, researchers Brian Day and Richard Fitzpatrick state that the vestibular system:

> ...provides our brains with a deep and special understanding of how the force of gravity moves things, from the fall of our body as we lift our foot to take a step, to the fall of a ball during a game of cricket. In all of these situations, the brain predicts the trajectory of fall with startling accuracy.

We understand how gravity affects objects because we first understand how gravity affects our own bodies; from the increased muscle action needed to control our head balanced on top of our neck, to the feel of horizontal movement when we're being carried versus vertical movement as we are set down, to the coordination of our eyes and ears around our center as we rotate left and right. All these sensations must match up accurately and consistently to build a database of vestibular sensory experiences that allows us to translate our experiences into guesses about how gravity affects other people and things.

As our brains plan a **motor action**, they also make another set of plans about the results of that action. This second set of plans, called reafference, tells the brain what to expect in response to our motor movement, it connects the dots between a physical force and the subsequent reaction. This constant communication between vestibular input, motor output and skeletal muscles creates the smooth and controlled movements we can make, responding quickly to increase or decrease muscular force as we interact with our physical environment.

If you add in interaction with the frontal lobe of the cerebrum (which helps us project the consequences of our actions) and the muscles of the eyes, this creates what is termed **feedforward**; the ability to anticipate a movement and move accordingly. When a ball is thrown to you, to catch it you don't put your hand out at the height at which you first saw the ball in your visual field. You anticipate a drop in the ball's height as it travels, and move your hand to where the ball *will be* when it reaches you. That's feedforward. In this example, it's easy to see where that chain of events could break down if your vestibular system wasn't always providing you with accurate information about gravity, weight and force.

Your guess about the projected course of the ball would be difficult to trust.

If you think of this difficulty with the feedforward loop in terms of behavior, children with these difficulties cannot "guess" what might happen when they take certain action. For the ball example above, a child's reaction may be to cover their face in response to a ball chucked toward them, even if that ball was not traveling in the direction of their face. Some children will impulsively enact each idea they have to satisfy their curiosity about the result of their action. These children do seemingly irrational things, making us ask in frustration, "What were you thinking?!" The answer is, "I didn't know what was going to happen, so I had to try it," but children often cannot articulate this.

When children with feedforward dysfunction come in to the clinic, often they persist in playing with a toy designed for much younger children, long after that toy should have lost its appeal for them. A particular toy in my office has holes just the right size to hammer a ball through, then watch it travel down a series of short ramps to the bottom. If a child is older than about two years, it is developmentally appropriate that this toy should pique their interest, but then quickly be abandoned as they figure out it doesn't do much else. If this toy is their favorite during each session in my toy-filled room—if they never seem to tire of it—then I know they may not easily understand the physical consequences of their actions. They continue to play with this toy because it is "new" every time. They don't know that the stationary ramp will always cause the ball to roll with the same speed and direction. A toy like that is fun for everyone, but the age-appropriate response after the age of two should be, "Well, I've got that figured out. What's next?" If a child 'stuck' on this toy loses interest in it, I know we have made therapeutic progress.

Mechanisms of Dysfunction

While we can't know if a child's multiple ear infections actually contributed to dysfunction, there is some evidence to support the idea. Recall that the brain is wiring very fast in childhood. If a misconnection is made, and not pruned because accurate information is never received, that misconnection can remain, and even strengthen. A 2001 study by Bennett et al. found that certain repeated ear infections in early childhood have been correlated with hyperactive and inattentive behavior up to the age of 15 years, and also with decreased reading ability between 11 and 18 years.

Deaf children have a much higher incidence of ADHD than the general population; as high as two-to-three times higher in deaf children than hearing children. But more subtle, less-detectable ear dysfunction can also impact behavior. In a 2013 study by Antoine et al., on mice in which vestibular function had been chemically compromised, researchers found that the severity of vestibular impairment could result in different behaviors. More profoundly impaired mice manifested hyperactive behaviors, while less severely impaired mice exhibited signs of anxiety. This could be analogous to the difference between a child who has a severe and lingering ear infection at a developmentally-crucial stage of development, who later develops ADHD, compared with a child who has chronic low-level middle-ear fluid retention due to allergies, and later struggles with learning and reading or is overly anxious.

The study mentioned above focuses on the severity of the deficits within the vestibular system. There are many other structures of the body and brain that contribute to physical responses; narrowing it down to just one system and collection of neurons may be an oversimplification. But, at least in mice, we can study other factors that may be influencing behaviors related to vestibular function. A 2009 study compared the behavior of adult mice who had their vestibulae removed to mice that had their vestibulae removed before birth (Baranek and Lambert). For the adult mice, who once had a functional vestibular system, there was a transitory period of positional disorientation and coordination problems. Then the mice recovered near-normal function, in an excellent illustration of neural plasticity. For the mice born without a functional vestibular system, there were permanent impacts on their behavior, such as constant circling and disorientation. This led the researchers to conclude that the period of development in which damage to vestibular function occurs can alter the coordination and navigation capacities of the mice, and perhaps humans as well.

It is incredibly difficult to definitively say that impaired vestibular function results in certain behaviors. The brain can recover lost function through neural plasticity, the severity of vestibular deficits can be variable, and the period of development in which damage occurs can impact function. There are lots of neurological processes that occur between vestibular input and motor output. It is impossible to predict which behaviors will occur for which children. It is not even possible to predict what outcomes can be obtained through regimented vestibular therapy. But in my years of practice, I have seen so many positive behavioral changes happen during the course of controlled vestibular therapy, and the connection between the two cannot be coincidental, in my opinion. Because of the brain's surprising ability to re-wire itself, given the right input, I advocate that every neurodiverse child go through a trial period of vestibular treatment. The brain is so flexible, that to withhold the possibility of improvement through this type of therapy seems unfair.

One of my favorite illustrations of our flexible and adaptable neural wiring comes from the book *Fixing My Gaze* by Dr. Susan Barry. The book tells the story of how Dr. Barry achieved binocular vision (seeing three-dimensionally) after a lifetime of strabismus. Because her eyes did not act in concert when she was a child, her brain adapted by seeing through one eye at a time, the result being that she only ever saw the world two-dimensionally. But in her forties, Dr. Barry was treated by a developmental optometrist. Through a series of prescribed exercises, she was able to see in three dimensions and her visual world gained depth.

While her story is itself an excellent example of neural plasticity in an adult, the more illustrative story regarding vestibular function actually comes from her husband, Dan. Dan is a NASA astronaut and he spent a week in space, in an environment in which his vestibular system could not tell him anything about his position and where "down" was. After his trip, his daughter decided to run a few experiments on him at home. She asked him to close his eyes and raise his arm directly up. He was off by 60 degrees. She asked him to sit on his bed, then walk to the bathroom with his eyes closed. Despite making this trip in the dark countless times, Dan ran into the dresser. She asked him to close his eyes and stand on one foot; he immediately fell over. Of course, in a few days Dan had re-adjusted to Earth's gravity and was fine. But after having only spent a few days in a gravity-free environment, his adult, fully-formed vestibular system had rewired, and his internal sense of his body and his position in the space around him was altered.

If change can happen so rapidly in the adult neurological system, how much more easily must a child's neurological system change? The good news is, although negative change can happen if the vestibular system is compromised, given the correct input to alert and normalize the vestibular system, children can begin to organize themselves. Knowing how gravity and movement should feel, through purposeful, regimented exposure to movement can increase their ability to feel safe and secure, divide their attention appropriately, coordinate their bodies and eyes, regulate themselves, and communicate with others.

7   Ground Zero

One of the most important functions of the vestibular system is to provide information about whether we are moving or not. When we *know* we are not moving, our brains label our location as the zero-point around which we orient ourselves. When we are moving, the vestibular system provides information which helps the brain calculate a new zero-point based on our speed, trajectory, and whether or not we are generating the movement ourselves, or experiencing movement from some force outside ourselves. In this chapter, we'll explore how the vestibular centers in the brain connect the vestibulae in our ears to the skeletal muscles of our bodies through the cerebellum, the part of the brain that coordinates bodily movement. In turn, the muscles of our bodies give feedback to the cerebellum, but also directly to the vestibular end organs themselves. This feedback loop allows you to realize when your head is at an angle, but your body is upright, which is perfectly safe, versus when your whole body, including your head, is leaning, which could be unsafe because it means you're falling.

Because the vestibulae sense the direction and nature of movement they are a key component in forming our point of view; the location from which we perceive the world. Understanding this point of view and how it moves with us when we move is essential to developing an understanding of our visual world, allowing us to recognize objects from different points of view, categorize them (because that is what the brain does) and learn how they function. Early-development researchers Gopnik, Meltzoff, and Kuhl artfully refer to this as the "External World Problem" that every baby must solve to make sense of their world. I can't possibly improve on their description of the essence of this problem:

"We don't even really see things in the room... The brown, bounded shape we think of as the table perpetually changes its form as we move around it. The apparently solid three-dimensional spoons and pepper mills are really just flat surface images on our eyes. The feel of the spoon in our hands is quite different from the shape we see. The surface of the table is full of discontinuities: white holes where it is hidden by plates and bowls... We seem to know about a world of objects with properties that are quite independent of us, a world of tables and spoons and healthy soup. But all we experience directly is an endlessly changing chaotic flow of sensations. This is the External World problem" (p. 5).

It might be difficult to imagine *not* having this most basic understanding of the world from your own point of view, but you can guess that it would be debilitating. You might not be able understand the world beyond simple sensations; you might only understand how things look or sound or feel, but have no idea of their purpose. Items and actions would have no context or meaning, and your world would be a disconnected chaos of feelings, sights and sounds. I believe this is the scattered existence in which some children live, particularly those with **profound autism**. It's really no wonder that a child without a sense of self cannot assign a purpose to that puzzle piece you just handed him. The concept of a "puzzle" and a "puzzle piece" cannot be built without a consistent perceptual point of view. So, what does he do with the puzzle piece I just handed him? Well, sensation is all he has to work with, so experiencing the sensation of this thing he can't name or categorize allows him only so many choices: the visual sensation of spinning on the table, the sound of slapping it on his palm, or the taste of chewing on it.

Without the understanding of perspective, children might also have a difficult time understanding the size or magnitude of objects. They might fail to appreciate that something they can hold in their hands is smaller than they are, or where they fit in a large space, like a house. Understanding the size of something you don't physically touch is understood through auditory scene analysis and vision, but those have to be partnered with knowledge of movement. One uses all three systems (the auditory, vestibular and visual systems)

When a Child Doesn't Understand Size and Location

My little friend Courtney suffered from great anxiety during bath time because she was sure that her bath toys would travel down the drain with the water when the plug was pulled. No amount of showing her how they won't fit could ease her anxiety. Only when she began to have a sense of her center was she able to inherently understand the physics involved in something "not fitting" because of its size.

The lack of a perspective is also a potential explanation of unusual behavior of my friend's son, who has autism. Every time the family visited a friend's house, be it a familiar or new house, this boy went straight to the freezer. Every house had one, and this might have been his way of orienting to a space that was, in all other ways, incomprehensible to him. He oriented to the freezer: as long as he knew where that was in the house, he knew where he was in relation to it.

---

together to comprehend that, when objects become larger in the visual field, it is because you are *moving* toward them. Without the ability to match the knowledge of movement with the visual and sound image changes, the concept and approximation of size becomes difficult to learn.

Besides helping us to understand our unique perspective as a singular person in the world, the vestibular system helps us build a sense of our center of gravity. Children without an accurate vestibular sense have difficulty assigning a center of gravity to objects because they don't know where their own center of gravity is located. They have trouble making motor plans that involve objects, so they always seem to be trying to do things that are physically impossible. For example, in my clinic, when a child sees a row of three blocks stacked on top of a row of four blocks, they will try to replicate it by beginning to stack two blocks together on top of one, and not quite understanding why that doesn't work.

In the book *The Scientist in the Crib*, the authors postulate, and give evidence, that "[babies] and young children think, observe and reason. They consider evidence, draw conclusions, do experiments, solve problems and search for truth" (p.13). If a child has faulty or inconsistent data during their experiments, they could be repeating the same experiments *ad nauseum*, because the satisfying conclusion of "figuring it out" can't be reached. Figuring out how objects of different masses interact requires an estimation of their centers of gravity. The physics of a game like billiards is an excellent example. Predicting how the force and trajectory of one ball will affect another is an extension of our understanding of where our own center of gravity is located, and then projecting that idea onto an object. That can only happen effectively for people who receive accurate vestibular information.

Children who cannot easily assign a center of gravity, and therefore a very specific location in space, to themselves, will also have trouble assigning a different point in space as the location for a completely separate person. Children who lack this internal sense of where they are located in space may have a hard time with body boundaries and thinking of themselves as separate from objects or other. Autism-activist and author Temple Grandin explains that "people with autism sometimes have body boundary problems. They are unable to judge by feel where their body ends and the chair they are sitting on or the object they are holding begins" (p. 25).

This difficulty with separation of self from others would also impede solving another problem that crib-scientists encounter; the "Language" problem. To understand that these funny sounds coming out of another person's mouth are an attempt to communicate something, a child must first understand that *their* thoughts and *that person's* thoughts are different, because they are different people who occupy a different space. This may be why **language develops** *after* a child psychologically establishes that a parent, usually Mom, is a completely different person. This usually manifests itself in the form of separation anxiety around nine months of age, and language develops around a twelve to fourteen months.

If a child doesn't consider another person as separate from them (and this especially applies to Mom and Dad) why would he need to communicate what he is thinking? The other person already knows! I actually consider it a good developmental step when a parent reports to me that their five- or six-year-old child lies to them for the first time. Lying is a normal stage of development for a two- or three-year-old, and if a child is six and has never lied, it indicates that they might not appreciate that others are separate being with

> ### Perspective and Non-verbal Communication
> Higashida also lacks a sense of his unique position in space. He writes that he persisted in waving good-bye to others with his palm facing him. That was his perspective when others waved to him, and he didn't understand that others were seeing his action from *their* perspective.

separate viewpoints and knowledge, and therefore can be hoodwinked through false information.

Because of this difficulty sensing boundaries between themselves, objects or other people, some children will become upset beyond reason to see *someone else* breaking the rules, or doing something they dislike. I believe it is because their sense of where they are in space is not sufficiently telling them they are NOT where the other person is, and are not experiencing what the other person is experiencing. This skill is normally evident in three-year-olds, who can hide a toy from an examiner by placing it on *their* side of a screen, not the examiner's, or understand that *you* might like broccoli, while *they* like crackers.

We have all watched someone perform an action we might view as revolting, such as watching a surgeon reaching into someone else's body during a medical procedure, and had the reflexive reaction of "Ew, gross!" That response is very functional. It develops empathy for another person because we can imagine what it is like to be in their shoes. However, if we need to continue to function, we must not become overwhelmed. We look away, we mentally distract ourselves, or we remind ourselves of that what we are feeling is not what the other person is feeling. Maybe we even take a moment to feel our own bodies more closely to establish more concretely that we are ok, such as when we take deep breaths. For children without an adequate sense of the space they occupy, that distinction becomes difficult to make, and watching someone perform an action is too closely related to doing the action themselves.

Staying Grounded

Because the vestibular system provides information about our zero-point, it is a primary factor in staying oriented within our bodies and within the situation. I refer to it as 'staying grounded'. Recall the four arenas of time and space through which we move functionally, all day long—mental space, far space, near space and body space. Knowing where we are in the physical body and in the situation at hand allows us the freedom and control to move between mental and physical spaces as necessary to accomplish tasks. Placing our point of perspective precisely where we are within our surroundings accurately, in both time and space, allows us to interact effectively with physical objects, plan our immediate actions, and maintain our attention within a sequence of events. A functional person is mentally present within the timeline of their day, which allows them the ability to sequence events. One's internal dialog might be something like this: "We are leaving the house for a shopping trip in a few minutes. Have I brushed my teeth? Nope, gotta do that and put on some makeup before we leave. Oops, can't forget the shopping bags!"

Children who aren't grounded in their bodies may visually lock onto anything stationary because it gives them an orientation in space and helps them feel secure, but this can keep them trapped in near space. I have worked with children who will play, seated or lying on the floor, with any toy you give them, and not really object when that toy is switched to a new toy, as long as the toy is in the same location. It is my presumption that these children cannot inherently sense their position in space independently and accurately, so relating the location of their body to the location of the toy helps them stay grounded in place.

Other children might depend on the proprioceptors in their muscles and joints to provide information about staying upright. But this information varies with external factors, like the nature of the surface one is standing on, what one is carrying, or even if one is exposed to a strong wind. All of this changes the proprioceptive feedback to our muscles and the information provided by a functional vestibular system is what coordinates all that sensory information to keep the body upright, safe and oriented.

Children who depend on their proprioceptive system to stay oriented are usually in **constant movement**. This activity provides lots of chances to become more coordinated at moving, running and jumping. A child's high level of coordination could mistakenly give the impression that the vestibular system is working and communicating well with the body and brain. But these children are likely to have fine motor deficits, be hyper-emotional or rigid in their thinking, or have difficulty learning mental concepts. They may struggle to fall asleep at night and sleep very little. Often in these cases, parents don't seek out help for their child until they are school age and this behavior starts to impede their ability to learn.

I see this pattern often in children who are **early walkers,** starting to walk at 9 months or so, or children who skip crawling altogether and go from sitting to cruising and walking. These children require a larger-than-normal intensity of movement for vestibular input to register, as well as increased input to their muscles and joints, in order to feel safe. So, they begin bearing weight and moving around their environment as early as possible because it feels better and more grounding to move in big ways. However, their vestibular system is still dampened and does not provide adequate feedback when they are stationary. Again, Naoki Higashida, gives us insight into how this feels; "When I'm not moving, I feel like my soul is detaching itself from my body, and this makes me so jumpy and scared that I can't stay where I am" (p. 106)

Taking It All Off

Vestibularly-challenged kids are looking for additional information from their environment to help them stay oriented, and for some children that can mean adding the feeling of surfaces to their tactile sensors by removing their shoes or clothing. This can happen at very inopportune times, and it's one of the signs I would like to see improve early on in treatment. As a child's sense of vestibular awareness improves, they may continue to like to **remove their clothes or shoes,** but I often find that within the first month or two of treatment, they can "deal" with situations like being in public without removing clothing, and the family can enforce a "naked is for home only" policy.

Knowing Where "Down" Is

The primary area of the vestibulum affecting our sense of where "straight down" is, and therefore where our center of gravity is, is the saccule. The saccule is stimulated in an obvious way when your ride up or down on a fast-moving elevator. Your eyes tell you the world is stationary, but you feel that moment, as the elevator begins to move up, that you "feel" heavier. As inertia settles in, this sensation lessens. As an aside, I think this may contribute to why some perfectly rational adults fear elevators; the sensory mismatch.

In my occupational therapy work with children, understanding the saccule is crucial because so many of our physical interactions with the world depend on our innate knowledge of where "directly down" is. Knowing when our head or limbs are off-center from "down" allows our brain to calculate their weight and create points of comparison for forces required to interact with the physical world. The saccule is like a carpenter's plumb line, shifting to keep track of which direction is down no matter how our bodies shift, giving us this information to match up with which muscles need to contract to keep us upright and safe. Children don't have as much experience as adults interacting with the physical world. They are constantly doing things for the first time in their lives. They need the vestibular system to be giving them consistent, accurate information so that they can learn to make all the necessary adjustments for how much force to use—through which muscles and in which direction— to complete a task; from picking up a glass of water to giving a hug.

If the saccule is not accurately sensing which direction is straight down, a child will have a hard time knowing the weight and center of gravity of objects, and therefore have difficulty sensing how much force will be necessary to perform a task. This sense of gravity's effect on the body creates a point of comparison for guessing gravity's effects on objects, and therefore how to physically interact with them; to calculate how much force to use to lift or move a given object.

Neurotypical babies explore their own center of gravity as they begin to hold their head upright, and as they learn to sit unsupported. Shortly after these milestones, they begin to play with the effect of gravity of the objects around them. How many times will a baby throw its rattle off the edge of the high chair tray? As many times as it takes to learn how hard it needs to be pushed to get over the edge and that the rattle will always go down.

But there are some people, as explained by Naoki Higashida, for whom earth's gravity doesn't feel strongly *enough*. He created a character in one of his stories called Autisman, who prefers to live on his home planet where gravity is heavier, because in earth's gravity he always feels as if he is "swimming in space, weightlessly" (p. 46).

The plumb-line of the saccule also helps develop **body scheme.** Learning right and left, internal and external, and front and back within the body happens only when one knows where the center is, and orients to that. Knowing where our center is allows us to develop our internalized "body map." A great example of how we know our body's scheme is represented in the oral-motor control required for eating. Biting, chewing and swallowing involve fine motor movements that are developed strictly through a sense of touch and proprioception. We can't monitor the movement of our mouths with our eyes. A child who isn't grounded in their body, who doesn't have an accurate plumb-line, may not be able to know how to move food forward and back within their mouths. The motions of chewing or the location of food within the mouth cannot be visually monitored and may not be sensed strongly or accurately. Manipulating food, tasting food, and coordinating chewing, swallowing and breathing might require a level of attention that is difficult for a child with little sense of their internal world.

Always in Threat Mode

When children don't understand how gravity affects them and their bodies, they feel insecure or disconnected from the world . Being disoriented and "off-balance" at baseline means that these children may have strong emotional and physiological reactions. These children can seem emotionally hypersensitive, or be unable to tolerate new or slightly uncomfortable sensations. They may feel threatened by sensations that other children can tolerate because of the vestibular center's direct connection with the tenth cranial nerve, the vagal nerve. The vagal nerve influences our response to stressors in our environment, our "fight or flight" response. It has connections to the gastrointestinal tract (and therefore vomiting), the esophagus, the voice box, the diaphragm and other breathing muscles (and hyperventilation) and the cardiac control mechanisms. The vagal nerve may be persistently in high-alert mode already and may play a significant role for those kids with picky eating habits, whose responses to just seeing or smelling a noxious food involve a gag response and vomiting.

Without a central plumb line, a child's internal world might be so disorganized that they are not able to tune into their body. They may not be familiar with sensations like hunger and satiety. This can compound the problem of **picky eating** because the hunger that creates the drive to eat slightly unappealing foods is not present. And because a child might already be in heightened state of threat, they are unable to accept new foods as non-threatening because they can's process the new sensations. I remember the first time I had a fizzy drink, like soda. I wasn't expecting such a strong sensation, and it was weird to feel the fizz, even up into my sinuses. It was strong, and odd, but not bad. Because I was oriented in my body, the sensations that were new and different were not threatening. There was no gagging, and there was a willingness on my part to try it again, now that I knew better what to expect. This level of processing can happen for picky eaters too, once they are oriented to their place in time and space and can pay attention to the sensations in their body without anxiety.

Research Zinc

Low oral awareness sometimes involves the sense of taste as well as pressure sensors and muscles within the mouth. If your child doesn't request specific foods, prefers very strong flavors, or doesn't get excited about eating, their **sense of taste** may not be strong enough. All food may taste the same—bland. That greatly decreases anyone's desire to eat. One potential solution is to explore adding really strong flavors (citrus, salt, pepper, etc.) to neutral-tasting foods and see how your child responds. Another avenue is to explore the possibility that your child may be low in zinc, the mineral that is essential to the firing of our taste sensors. There is a test called zinc-tally that is commercially available and will give you an opportunity to see if this is an issue for your child. Zinc supplements are also available. Do some research—Google is your friend here.

Kevin Puts it All Together

When a child becomes more connected with the center of their body their coordination improves, they handle disruptions better emotionally, they communicate more easily, and they seem more at home in their bodies. These are all wonderful changes that I see in the clinic, but are very difficult to communicate in the pages of a book. However, my friend Kevin was kind enough to provide a superb visual illustration of the changes that can happen when a child gains a sense of their body by having a center point around which to build it.

When I met Kevin, he was nine-years-old, but he was unable to answer simple questions about where he lived, couldn't follow directions with multiple steps, had only recently learned to dress himself and seemed very anxious. He apologized throughout his evaluation for not being able to complete tasks before he'd even attempted them. His mother reported that he was born via emergency c-section and had over 20 ear infections in his early childhood. He had had it rough! She wanted him to be more independent, mentioning that he needed someone's company and attention (usually hers) during every hour of the day. His ocular-motor function was very limited and seemed to be that impacting his academic abilities; he was skipping letters when writing his name and had illegible handwriting.

One of the tasks I have almost every child do when I meet them is draw a picture of themselves. While there is a formal test called the Draw-a-Person Test, my evaluations typically include a more casual request for a child to draw me a picture of themselves. During his evaluation, this drawing task seemed to stymie Kevin. He initially drew a television, which told me that he might be a child who orients himself to things around him instead of to his own body. When I asked him to add himself to the picture, this is what he drew (even adding the arrow toward the TV) as shown in Fig. 7-1 on the next page.

Kevin was doing the best he could, but his orientation in space was very poor, perhaps contributing to his anxiety and need for his mother's attention. His spatial skills were impaired, limiting his ability to move his eyes, and therefore read and write. His body awareness was non-existent and he had been keeping himself oriented by latching onto objects visually, like his TV.

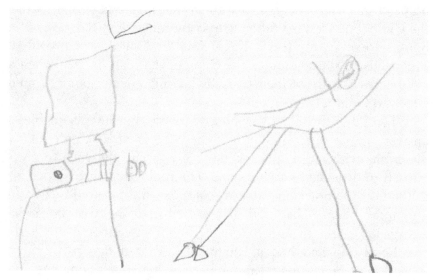

Fig. 7-1: Kevin's self-portrait February 26.

As his treatment (which was both auditory and vestibular) pro-gressed, he was better able to follow directions, and had improved his balance, reading and writing. He was more confident moving around and trying new things. But the strong change in his body-perception was graphically displayed in this drawing (Fig. 7-2), which he made a few months later. His handwriting on the page is legible, he is alone on the page, and he has all his body parts—even his heart is in the right place!

I believe that tactile and movement interventions are less effective without corresponding treatment to increase vestibular awareness. The connection between body awareness and vestibular function may not be obvious. In treatment, common sense would dictate that stimulating different parts of the body through movement and touch would help to increase body awareness. In my experience, those things *do* help. But I also find that, if a child has no "ground-zero" to relate those new sensations to, then the increase in awareness remains unrelated to where they are in space and how gravity affects them.

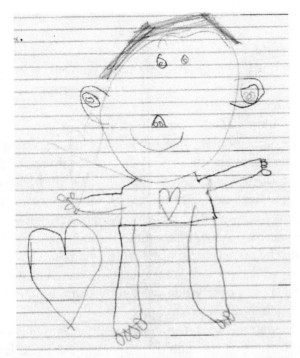

Fig. 7-2: Kevin's self-portrait August 12, same year.

When a child feels off-balance, as if they cannot trust that the ground beneath them will hold them up, it's very hard to commit their attention elsewhere. Therefore, it takes a stronger stimulus than it should for a child's brain to register a sensation.

As we'll explore in the next chapter, this lack of attention can have an impact on behaviors that don't seem related to moving or sensing movement. Paying attention to internal sensations like body scheme, proprioception, hunger and thirst, even the need to use the bathroom, are all more difficult when a child has no vestibularly-provided sense of center. That center is a very small point at the core of our bodies and it's the zero-point from which our sense of our bodies, and then our sense of the world beyond our bodies, develops.

The Vestibular-Vision Connection

Observing a child's eye movements can be a good indicator of their vestibular function. Can they look at me? Can they follow an object across their visual field? If they are an older child, do they have difficulty with reading? Do they look up, in the correct direction, to an unexpected noise? In a previous chapter, we explored auditory function's role in locating things visually in the environment. But there is a second necessary component to locating things in the environment; one that is dependent on the vestibular system. Before a child can orient toward a stimulus in the environment, they must first know where *they* are.

The vestibular centers directly connect to the **extraocular muscles**. The extraocular muscles are six muscles per eye that control the movement of the orb of the eye within the skull, allowing our eyes to look up, down, to the side, and all the variations in between. These are very sensitively calibrated muscles that make micro-movements, every day, all day throughout our lives. Jumping movements from one visual image and location to another are called *saccades*, and they occur most noticeably when our eyes jump from word to word while we read. Smoother, larger movements are called *pursuits*, and these occur when we follow something through our visual field, such as a car driving past.

These movements alternate all day to allow us to visually take in important information through the camera of our eyes. Just like an actual camera, for the image to be stable, the eyes must be on a stable base. Not only a base that is stationary and can move the camera's focus around at will, but one that compensates for movement of that base (our bodies) as *it* moves through space.

The vestibular system has direct connections to the muscles of the eyes and neck, so that eye movement and stability can be rapidly responsive. For example, when we are walking, our extraocular muscles compensate for the up-down motion of our heads with each step. This happens through a communication between the extraocular muscles and the vestibular system called the Vestibular Ocular Reflex. For extraocular muscles to develop properly, vestibular sensory information about movement and stillness must be consistent and reliable from moment-to-moment and from day-to-day. If a child has ocular-motor difficulties, it is may be that this consistent, reliable vestibular information was not always available.

Many occupational therapists look at one specific involuntary eye reflex, called **nystagmus**, which can be elicited through movement, as an opportunity to observe the vestibular system's function. Nystagmus is the occurrence of the eyes moving repetitively across the visual field, without voluntary intent from the brain.

For a neurotypical person, spinning around 10 times *should* create a nystagmus response, lasting for about 10 to 20 seconds before settling down. Once we become dizzy in this way, the world seems to go on spinning, visually, even though we have stopped. This occurs because the fluid in the semicircular canals of the vestibular system is still moving, due to inertia, when the spinning stops. Once the fluid in the semicircular canal settles, the nystagmus response should pass. However, in some children, the nystagmus response is weak or nonexistent, sometimes indicating an under-responsive vestibular system or a weak connection between the vestibular system and the muscles that control visual direction.

A typical nystagmus response illustrates the rapid, very strong connection between the eye muscles and the vestibular system. This is necessary for functional, smooth movement that is visually guided. The vestibular system plays an integral role in our navigation through the world and our mental map of our surroundings. Just like the screen on a car's GPS, our mental map can rotate in our mind as our eyes swing through the environment. But the map's orientation can only align with the way we view the world visually if we have a very accurate and sensitive gauge for how far we move our head and eyes in any direction.

The vestibulae are in a fixed position within the head. They can only sense when the *head* is moving in a given direction. Imagine

---

Using Nystagmus as an Indicator

Clinicians and researchers disagree regarding the therapeutic importance of the strength and duration of nystagmus. The factor to which I pay attention clinically is the presence or absence of the response. Achieving a present and normally-sustained nystagmus response in a child who had none at evaluation is an informal therapy goal in my treatment, simply because it indicates new or strengthened neural connections between the vestibular sensors and ocular-motor muscles. If the eyes and the vestibular system are in communication, the eyes are more likely to provide a stable visual image to the brain during tasks like walking and running, which increases coordination. In a study of four-year-old children, those with no post-rotary nystagmus performed consistently worse on motor tests than children with normal post-rotary nystagmus response (Mailloux et al., 2014).

your brain is the 'driver' of a 'car' that is your body. The front of the car (your body) can be moving in one direction (north, east, west, south) at a time. But the driver (your brain) observing the world from within the car must have a wider scope than strictly straight ahead. The driver must anticipate obstacles and plan routes independent of the direction of the car's trajectory, but still coordinating its movements. Your brain is able to separate the motions of your head (to scan the environment) and the motions of your body (to move forward).

To do this, information from the vestibulae travels along two different, simultaneous tracts. One tract sends messages to the neck and core muscles and cerebellum, where it is combined with incoming messages from the muscles of the body, to create a frame of reference for movement. A second tract, creates a second frame of reference that accommodates for movements of the mind-map that match the rotation of the eyes within the skull (Angelaki and Cullen, 2008). For this mind-map to move accurately, it must sense eye motions and head motions down to single degrees, so the difference between moving your head five degrees to the right, or your eyes ten degrees to the left, can shift the mind-map accordingly, and you can stay oriented. With such a delicately calibrated system, one can imagine that too much movement, such as spinning excessively, could throw the system out of whack for a moment or two. That normal response when the system goes out-of-whack is nystagmus.

Using Substitutions Changes Behavior

A child's preferred method of substituting for the vestibular information they are missing, visual, proprioceptive, or a combination of the two, can result in some specific behaviors that give us clues about the information their brain is using. If a child is using their visual system to anchor themselves in space, they may not like lying down or looking down, keeping their head upright when picking things off the floor instead of looking down. They may be so dependent on *things* in the environment being upright (faces, doorways, etc.), to tell their brain that *they* are upright, that they don't want to tilt their head and take away this anchor. As an experiment, the next time you're driving, tilt your head a few degrees to the left or right. You'll pull it back into upright very quickly because it's uncomfortable for your brain. While driving, our brains are very visually-dependent because we can't hear or feel the outside world in our little metal box on wheels. Our brain doesn't want us to do anything that makes processing input from the eyes more difficult.

For some children who heavily use their visual system to orient themselves in space, they don't really walk to their destination. It seems that they visually lock onto a target, then "fall" in that direction, catching themselves by stepping their feet in front of them. This "visual lock" for orientation means that they have difficulty moving their eyes to observe potential obstacles. They trip over the edge of the mats in my room, or over toys on the floor. Often, a child who regularly trips or is "clumsy" will be classified as having gross-motor problems, but in my experience, it's just as likely, if not more so, that they have ocular-motor difficulties stemming from incomplete or inaccurate vestibular information. In the coming chapter, we'll explore other behaviors that may, in part, have a vestibular explanation.

A Little Hint

If your child uses his vision to stay oriented, tipping his head back to wash his hair can be a bit disorienting. Add to that the inability of vestibularly-challenged children to predict what will happen accurately, and suddenly they don't trust that you won't pour that water over their face and eyes, which doesn't feel very good. Bottom line: It's scarier than it should be.

---

8 What is Going On In There?

When the vestibular system is telling us that we are physically safe and stable, it allows our brain to perform one of its most imperative functions: ignoring stuff. Generally, we tend to think of our brains as paying attention or not paying attention. But attention is like a filter, it can get clogged with irrelevant information if those stimuli aren't removed from the stream. Our brains remove unimportant information by ignoring it through the process of habituation. A stimulus may have caught our attention, for example the feel of the chair under our bum as we sit down. As we remain sitting, we no longer need that input. We *know* we're sitting—our attention is needed elsewhere. But if our vestibular system isn't providing us with the feeling of dependable stability, it may feel safer for our brain to stay keyed into that bum-input, to *make sure* we're stable. But now there's less space in our attention-filter for learning.

The Reticular Formation

Attention is a prime example of how the vestibular system can influence behaviors that don't appear to be at all related to balance and movement. Vestibular input helps the brain to decide what sensations should be raised to conscious attention. The brain decides what information makes it thorough the filter using a complex network of neurons called the **reticular formation**. The reticular formation is the gateway that affects attention and levels of arousal; on a continuum from a hyper-aroused state of fight-or-flight, to extremely focused in an adaptive state of being "in the zone", to being in a completely "unplugged" state, such as meditation or sleep. In each of these situations, a functional reticular formation filters what information comes into our consciousness. When a person is afraid they will fall, they may not be able to process what is being said to them, or when they are lying securely asleep, they can ignore sound and movement in the environment that would normally catch their attention.

The connection between the vestibular system and the reticular formation contributes greatly to the process of habituation. Like the auditory system, when sensory matches are continually made between the vestibular sense and other sensory systems, the information gets filtered out of our consciousness. If we feel the chair under our bottom and the floor under our feet, and our center of gravity feels securely over our base of support, and all this matches with the vestibular sensation that we are upright and unmoving, then the feel of the chair and floor, and other sensations like the clothes on our skin and our minute muscle contractions can be filtered out.

In a situation in which there is a sensory mismatch, however, much more sensory information floods into the brain. The reticular formation realizes it might need conscious help from the upper brain centers to decide what is safe and what is not. So it "lets in" information about what the body is feeling, just in case it is relevant. This information then absorbs a portion of our available attention to sift through and interpret. That leaves less and less attention available for daily functions, learning and building relationships.

This dysfunctional relationship may play out behaviorally something like this: To feel physically secure, a child's body will seek out additional information to answer the question, "Am I safe?" His body will decide that it is better and safer to just be on his feet and moving to receive muscular feedback from his legs. Because his brain is seeking out additional sensation from his body, he can sense that seam in his sock and his brain can't shut it out. It continues to take a portion of his attention, and may even create a situation in which he becomes frustrated or uncomfortable. Children who can not ignore or are strongly repulsed by tactile sensations (that other people can tolerate) are often labeled **tactilely defensive**.

Lacking a functional habituation process not only limits a child's ability to feel calm in his body, but it may impact his ability to feel mentally and emotionally calm as well. Things that are not inherently dangerous may carry an additional threat with them because they are unexpected surprises. Because he already does not feel physically secure and stable, emotional consequences such as tantrums and anxiety ensue.

Looking Through a New Lens

It might be helpful to look at a few fairly common behaviors among children I have treated. This will help you better understand the connection between behavior and inner ear function, but you might recognize specific behaviors that your own child struggles with. Keep in mind that auditory, vestibular and visual function make up a three-legged stool that supports daily behavior and function. Sometimes it's hard to discern which leg of the stool is causing a problem because they are so interrelated, so in treatment, it's most effective to address all three.

Sleep

Sleep is a very complex neurological process, but in essence, the body must shut-down and surrender to fall asleep. While asleep, the body must feel safe enough to stay in this suspended state so there is enough time for it to mend cells, process new emotions and thoughts from the day, and dream. The mind continues to be active, but the body must withdraw from activity. The disconnection of the thinking mind and the acting body happens through the action of the **Reticular Activating System** (RAS). The RAS is a part of the Reticular Formation, the neural network that connects our thinking brain with our acting bodies. The RAS in particular is responsible for modulating which messages from the body get to the brain and which messages from the brain get to the body. During sleep, the RAS is the gate-keeper, keeping us from acting out our dreams physically, and keeping us asleep despite regular, expected noises or movements, such as our spouse joining us in bed.

The auditory and vestibular systems continue to send information to the RAS throughout the night. The RAS must "decide" whether to let neural impulses from these systems rise to the level of consciousness and wake us up from our sleep. Once the RAS is active, it shuts down neural impulses to and from the body. To activate the RAS, the reticular formation must allow for the low level of arousal at rest that *precedes* sleep. Input from vestibular system can excite or calm the reticular formation. Exciting the reticular formation may occur through the movement associated with exercise; one reason why we're advised not to exercise before bed. However, vestibular input can also *calm* the reticular formation, and parents use this method all the time to soothe infants to sleep on a car ride or in a mechanical swing. In the absence of trustworthy vestibular data, the reticular formation might stay "switched on" to sensations it should habituate to and ignore, interfering with the potential for sleep.

If a child is not getting adequate sleep, it can affect every aspect of her function. It can affect family dynamics as the parents and other family members are also stressed from lack of sleep. A good night's sleep can be a game-changer for a child and her family. When vestibular therapy improves sleep within the first few weeks of treatment, I often find this out after the fact. Because parents don't initially understand the vestibular-sleep connection, they may not mention their child's lack of sleep as we begin therapy. But as we proceed in treatment, I'm pleased when parents report to me, "He slept through the night for this first time ever last night!" This is almost always said with a smile, and sometimes it means that Mom or Dad had their first full night of sleep in years.

If a child's vestibular system isn't sending adequate information about her position in space to create a feeling of safety, it becomes very difficult for the child to enter physical shut-down mode, assisted by the reticular formation. These children will stay up late and/or sleep little, but tend to be very heavy sleepers. Because they aren't physically or emotionally comfortable at rest, they have to keep going and going, until their body reaches shut down from sheer exhaustion. Then, they collapse into a deep sleep for a few hours.

These children are sometimes difficult to potty train because their body shuts down *all* sensations coming in so that they can sleep and recover. Staying dry through the night can be a challenge when a body enters as deep a level of sleep as theirs does to regain some level of function. Think about it. We close our eyes, taking away the visual cues that we are safe and still, and proceed to "fall" asleep, which requires complete relaxation of the skeletal muscles. If those muscles are providing feedback for the child to feel secure, then it would be scary to relax them completely.

Once they finally hit the wall and their body forces them to sleep, it might only be for 3-4 hours, then they wake up and can't return to sleep. They awaken because, after initially falling asleep, their exhausted bodies go into a deep, restorative sleep and their RAS severs the brain's ties with the body. After 3-4 hours, everyone's RAS brings them to active, dreaming sleep, called REM sleep that is thought to help the brain process events of the day and cement them as memories. The brain's arousal level rises slightly to participate in the dream. For children who become disoriented at rest however, their body overreacts and wakes them up. If they get up and give themselves the movement they crave, they will feel less disoriented, so they get out of bed to play, find a parent, or run around.

If the problem creating a sleep disturbance is more auditory in nature, it's likely that a child is having trouble assessing a noise using their sound database (what was that noise?), having trouble with sound localization (where was that noise?), or having hearing hypersensitivity (Why won't that noise stop?). In all three occurrences, that sound rises to consciousness even though there is no threat and the brain should already have made the determination that the stimuli is not a threat. But until the auditory issue is addressed, be it processing, localization or sensitivity, noise will continue to rise to the consciousness-level to be analyzed as safe, interrupting a child's sleep.

Anxiety

The vestibular and auditory systems have connections to the limbic system, the emotional center of our brain. To decide which incoming information is a potential threat, these systems must access the part of the brain that feels anxiety and fear. If the information is potentially threatening, then our emotional circuits get involved to prepare us for a physical response, and the emotional circuits related to upset or anxiety may get activated.

It can be difficult for an adult who cares for an anxious child to find a balance between easing their anxiety and explaining that there are indeed times when caution should be exercised. Some children have constant debilitating fears, and others have fears that pop-up less frequently, but are disproportional to the reason for anxiety. The anxiety limits the child's comfort, attention or experiences, leaving them missing something in their lives. Children with extreme or unreasonable **anxiety** may have a diminished capacity to monitor their environment using the early-warning system that their hearing should provide, or they have little sense of their own center of gravity and are unable to assign a center of

Of Mice and Kids

A 2010 study of mice who had experienced genetic manipulation of their vestibular system found that those mice experienced more anxiety and stress during space-related tests, such as mazes and being hung by the tail, than did mice without alteration to their vestibular function[1]. In essence, tasks that were upsetting or challenging to unaltered mice, stimulated anxious behavior in those mice without dependable vestibular input. For our little rodent friends, this connection between vestibular function and anxiety was also established in a 2017 study of their vestibular system[1]. This study found that the severity of vestibular dysfunction affected a mouse's presentation as anxious (less severe vestibular dysfunction) or hyperactive (more severe vestibular dysfunction). In essence, mice with the same physiological dysfunction (vestibular problems) had different behaviors based on the severity of the dysfunction. It has been my experience that children also can display different behaviors and personalities that may have a common root problem.

gravity to others or objects, and therefore they are unable to predict the simplest physical interactions, like when something is likely to fall and when it isn't. These possibilities for unpredictability leave them with the unsettled feeling that the world is an unstable, scary place. Often, the children I work with have some combination of the two issues, because both are connected to the inner ear.

Hyperactivity

When a child is a bit short on vestibular information, their brain may choose to use other sensory inputs to orient and organize themselves; primarily visual or proprioceptive input. Kids who prefer to use their body's proprioceptive system to help anchor them in space can't sit still, and might be the textbook "ADHD kid." They prefer to do desk work or eat standing up. They may be constantly on the move, but they often can't make coordinated or smooth contact with someone or something else. They may be **toe-walkers**, adding lots of physical input through their legs while narrowing their base of support and increasing the vestibular sensations of losing their balance.

Some children who lack consistent vestibular system information will toggle back and forth between the two alternate methods of anchoring themselves in space, vision and proprioception. While a proprioceptive-anchorer may be able to stay seated to complete a game or task by switching to a visual-anchoring method, when left to his choice, he will likely choose an active game. Often times, when this child makes up a game, the rules will often not make sense or it will become physically **dangerous or physically impossible** as the game continues and the child becomes less and less oriented in space. Conversely, a visual-anchorer is likely to choose a sit-down game or task, but will need their hands placed on the floor for support or will wrap their legs around the legs of a chair for stability. Given the opportunity, they can rise to the occasion of a gross-motor game. It may be uncoordinated or require additional time and practice to be successful, but it will be possible.

Some very impaired children are unable to sit still, even for a moment; unable to create a position of stability from which to view and interact with the world. Albert was one such child. At four-years-old, he had never spoken any words or engaged appropriately with toys. He did not make eye contact with anyone or follow directions. He was **always on the move**, but walked on his toes and tripped over objects, or even his own feet, quite often. He was physically dependent for all activities except eating finger foods and needed constant supervision to remain safe. His parents reported that their biggest struggle was keeping him out of trouble, which was difficult because his constant movement meant there was always some new object to explore, whether it was safe or not. They reported that keeping him safe was also difficult because he slept only a few hours each night. During my initial time with him he never sat down or stopped moving around the room. He tripped several times, walked on his toes, and did not participate in any activities.

The first challenge of treatment was to get Albert to participate without tackling him and holding him down. Our first several sessions were spent in the net swing, which he enjoyed. My goal was to provide him additional input in the "down" direction, to help him understand his center of gravity and hopefully not need to be moving at all times to feel secure. The last ten minutes of each session were an opportunity to (hopefully) use some of his new-found orientation to sit at the table with me and engage with a toy. Sitting for these ten minutes was initially very challenging for Albert. Adding a supportive chair with arms to give him boundaries to his space helped, and he was able to sit for ten minutes within only a few treatment sessions. However, his ability to focus on a toy and play with it appropriately took many months.

While I waited for Albert's skills to rise to the level where we could play and interact, there were encouraging signs. A month or two after we began therapy, he no longer tripped on objects or lost his balance when walking around the room. He no longer needed someone to hold his hand to walk down the hall at school, but could follow in line like everyone else. He was also more visually attentive, making brief eye contact when someone addressed him closely.

After three months, he was participating in dressing by holding out his limbs. He was looking at people speaking to him about 60% of the time. By seven months of treatment, he was moving his eyes willingly around the room to look for specific toys and interacting with others by passing objects back and forth. After a year of treatment, he was sleeping through the night, following some commands by gestures, such as coming over to put on his shoes if his mother held them up. He could sit to watch TV and for dinner. He was even participating in class more, clapping with the music during music class.

While that year of treatment was much longer than I would typically see a child, and his progress was slow, it did occur in regular increments. And the difference for his family between a child who was completely dependent for all activities and one who could participate in activities such as getting dressed and sitting for dinner was a big deal. An increased awareness of his vestibular system created a sense of stability and security that allowed him to be an active participant in his world. That sense of being in control and understanding what was going on in a given situation reduced his anxiety and frustration and his behavior improved.

Auditory function can also have an impact on activity level. Children who don't easily interpret their environment through sound have specific behaviors that mimic hyperactivity or lead to inattention. Explored earlier, poor sound localization can influence the direction of a child's attention. Their attention may be contin-

Toe-Walking

Mild to moderate **toe-walking** often improves in the children who receive vestibular treatment without directly addressing the legs with exercises or ankle-foot orthoses. This may be because the child no longer needs the additional sensation of "falling" in every direction to stay balanced. Imagine the two circles below are each a child's body viewed from above (the triangle represents the nose) and the stars are their center of gravity. If the star is smaller, because the base of support is small (just the toes), the child begins to fall in some direction with very little movement. If it takes a larger movement before falling, this may make the child uneasy because they never know when a loss of balance may occur. If they are creating a loss of balance intentionally, all the time, it may increase their sense of space and safety. One goal of vestibular therapy is to help them feel safe with the bigger star (their feet) under them.

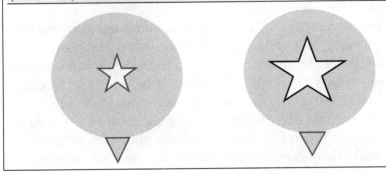

ually pulled away by irrelevant sounds they cannot filter out and might be potentially a threat. Or perhaps they are unable to isolate voices from background noise. These deficits can approximate the symptoms of what psychologists call ADHD, Inattentive Type. When a child can't use auditory scene analysis to know the size and scope of their space, they often will enter a new space and "make a lap." They will walk the perimeter of a new room, perhaps touching items along the way. Not only does this limit their ability to respond to what is relevant in the room, their need to be on the move looks a bit like hyperactivity. However, I find that this type of child, does just fine with stationary concentration once they are familiar with the room and it is just the two of us playing.

Picky Eating

The term '<u>picky eating</u>' can encompass a variety of behaviors. Some children become very emotional about trying new foods. Some children are labeled "stubborn" or "willful" over their difficulties eating what's provided. Some children simply are never hungry and don't tune into the sensations of their body. Gagging, vomiting and extreme emotional reactions are some of the cues I use clinically to help me separate out which children may be picky eaters because of a learned behavior, and which children are truly unable to tolerate new eating experiences because they are missing auditory or vestibular information. Children can sometimes be just as stubborn as adults. If a child simply doesn't want to eat a food because they don't like it, and whining and pouting are involved, that could just be an expression of a child's desire to not experience something they don't like. But, if a child will try a food, and it induces gagging or vomiting (even just once), or if the child is helpless with upset and fear at the idea of trying a food, then I attribute their picky eating to a potential physiological cause.

My reasoning is this: neither gagging, vomiting, or crying with fear is pleasant. If a child regularly chooses the unpleasant (and often exhausting) behaviors, as opposed to just trying a food, then I don't believe they are really "choosing" to behave as picky eaters. Food should not carry that high a threat-level for anyone. In treatment, I would like the child to have the tools to interpret the world safely and correctly (intact vestibular and auditory function), than to make them experience the threat over-and-over until it's less scary. It just seems kinder.

Picky eating may be a result of possible "breakdowns" in a child's orientation to their body and to the wider world. In the previous chapter, we explored breakdowns that may be auditory in nature, such as an inability or lack of experience with predicting the texture of a tactile experience based on how sound reflects off a surface.

When a child has a history of gagging and vomiting with certain foods, it's important for parents to understand the physiological reasons why a child might gag and vomit. When a child does not have a vestibularly-provided sense of their center of gravity, and therefore their specific, unique location in their environment, they may become upset just by seeing a reaction-causing food. Even watching other people eat a food they find noxious may make them anxious or upset, because they cannot separate themselves from another person in their mind easily. And perhaps because this lack of orientation in space creates a threat-response, the vagal nerve's connection to the vestibular system may even cause a gagging or vomiting reaction.

The feel of a specific food in their mouths creates a reflex reaction of physical anxiety that the food might be dangerous, and the resulting response is to eject it. This evolutionarily-constructed response protected our bodies in a time, historically, when food might have been rancid or might have appeared to be a safe food but was actually a poisonous look-alike plant or berry. Picky eating can be an issue for some children from birth; such as difficulty latching on when nursing as an infant, difficulty chewing once solid foods are introduced, or a lack of physical awareness of hunger. But for most picky eaters, they develop rejection of food around two or three years of age. In agrarian societies, this is the age in which a child would receive less supervision while a parent is in the field, and may well encounter things they might put in their mouths that look like food, but could be dangerous.

When the vestibular sense is working as it should, it gives us a feeling of spatial security and allows us the mental freedom to move our attention elsewhere, including to different places inside our bodies. Children who anchor to the world proprioceptively may be threatened because eating is almost always associated with sitting down. Some children may not be able to sit for long enough to eat a reasonable amount of food, or they may be so intent on staying moving and orienting themselves in exploration of their environment that they may not register a sensation of hunger, or a feeling a satiety tied to the act of eating. In a well-intentioned attempt to make sure their child is getting the nutrients they need, parents may leave food available at all times, allow constant "grazing" of snacks all day long, or supplement their child's intake with nutritional drinks. The problem with these approaches is that the child may not have a chance to feel true hunger, since the body sensation would need to be fairly strong to register with them, and then not have the opportunity to learn what action they can take (eating) to address that sensation. Remember, if the child doesn't use a neural connection, it gets pruned.

Also related to this lack of orientation to body sensations, is the lack of mental attention necessary to feel a food in the mouth and developmentally have the opportunities to create the neural connections that allow the exploration of the sensations of food without feeling threatened. Children with these challenges don't have the opportunity to increase their sense of safety by visually confirming what they are feeling and where objects are, because the food leaves their line of sight as it enters their mouths. They may not be able to know exactly when the food is going to touch their lips or mouth because they can't visually watch it happen, and their oral sensors and muscles may not be accurately feeling what is going on in their mouth. The entire process can be very threatening for children with low oral-motor and body awareness, and the result of that threat is often gagging and food rejection.

Children who are older but have a history of poor latching and feeding may still be struggling with the oral motor skills and timing of how to chew, breathe, move food around their mouths and swallow. That's a lot to accomplish when you're not sure if you might choke or not be able to breathe when your body tells you to. And those difficulties can be further compounded by a lack of oral motor skills and sensory awareness that can happen when a child doesn't have an accurate feeling of where they are and how their body feels.

Non-Food Chewing

If a child is a picky eater, their behavior regarding how they use their mouths tells me a lot. If they never explored with their mouths or mouthed toys as a baby, I tend to lean toward the possibility that their issues are more auditory in nature. If they constantly mouth non-food objects past infancy, I think they may be seeking stimulation to their midline to help them know where they are in space. These kids likely need our therapy to focus on vestibular input.

A word of advice to the parents of "chewers": if your child chews his sleeves, hair or the collar of his shirt, it might be a good idea to have her wear a chewing alternative. Sometimes these rubber "chewies" hang from a necklace or are worn like a bracelet. They are available from therapeutic supply companies and have names like Grabber, Chewelry and Munchables.

Tantrums

All children have challenging behavior sometimes. All children throw tantrums sometimes. But some families' lives are interrupted by <u>tantrums</u> that exceed the norm in either frequency or intensity, or both. Children with extreme tantrums have families that regularly change their plans or give up something to avoid a tantrum. Those tantrums may be a result of auditory or vestibular differences.

In my experience, children who have short, but intense or frequent tantrums may be having trouble with the auditory aspects of their environment. It may be as simple as being hypersensitive to the volume of noise in some situations, like the school cafeteria or a birthday party, and the tantrum may be an attempt to extricate themselves from discomfort. It may be, like my friend Paul in Chapter 3, that a child doesn't realize how long some tasks take, or are not oriented to time of day, so they are displeased when it is time to go to school and they are not done playing, or that they have to complete an unpleasant task and they don't know how little time it will actually take. Or perhaps a child doesn't understand another person's meaning in speech and they are frustrated by their inability to communicate. All these could be reasons for frequent tantrums that have an auditory source of dysfunction.

Sometimes challenging behaviors take the form of epic, seeming interminable or very physical tantrums. These tantrums are different. If there's any behavior that can affect a family more dramatically and regularly than epic tantrums, I don't know it. Tantrums can ruin trips to the park, big family events, and daily tasks like getting out the door to school. These tantrums are defined by their rapid onset, extreme physicality, possibly aggressive behavior, and long duration. Sometimes, the tantrum might continue after the child has been granted the thing they desire.

These tantrums usually begin when the child is diverted from their expected course of action. The child wants all objects and activities involved in her plan of action *exactly* the way she expects them to be. If the sequence, or color, or shape of the objects and activities don't match the image in her mind of what she expects, alarm bells ring in her head. I find that these children usually have more vestibular difficulties than auditory ones; although both can be present. Remember, vestibularly-challenged kids are already in a heightened state of alertness because their world is usually not secure and stable-feeling. They are trying their best to stay oriented in the time and space around them, but that often means preparing themselves for something coming up with cognitive effort, instead of being relaxed and adapting to events as they occur. To stay oriented, things must feel, look and be ordered as they were expecting, or else they are just plain wrong.

There is no "good enough" or "that will do fine" for some kids. A clue for me when I'm dealing with older children who suffer from these sensory mismatch challenges is that they are a bit compulsive about their schoolwork. Written work takes them quite a while because they are constantly erasing what they have written so that it looks just right. There are times that they get so hung-up on how their work looks, that they lose the object of the lesson and become quite frustrated.

Sometimes children who are having a tantrum can be physically aggressive with others. It can be frustrating for a parent who knows what a sweet, loving boy or girl their child is, to constantly hear about his or her misbehavior at school, or regularly have to

---

Thanks, Dad

When I was trying to "figure out" children who had epic tantrums, my dad was a great help to me. My father is a pilot and has flown all his life. I realize now that flying was his vestibular treatment. The vestibular stimulation and constant eye movement involved in flying helped him be more functional outside the cockpit; more grounded and adaptable to changes. Despite his self-treatment, he still struggles to adapt and recognizes that anger surfaces readily. He shared with me the following example of how his mind sometimes fails to adapt when things are not as he expects them to be: "When I am working under the car, and I reach for the wrench beside me, I get irritated if it's not where I was expecting it to be. If I have to reach a little further, I'm a little more irritated. If I have to reach a third time, or look around for it, I'm gonna be mad." I think the act of disengaging visually or mentally from "working on the car" to "finding the wrench" disorients him just enough that his less-than-oriented brain takes him straight to frustration and anger.

reprimand him or her for being aggressive with other children. The parent knows that the child's behavior doesn't reflect her true nature. The parent might be at a loss as to how to help their child reconcile *knowing* what is the kind and helpful thing to do is, with the behavior that seems to be beyond their control.

Angry, aggressive tantrums indicate that a child may be equally impaired in both the vestibular and auditory senses. Such profound impairments may explain why they become aggressive and stubborn in situations where other dysfunctional children might withdraw or try their best to meet the expectations of adults. So little about their physical bodies keeps them oriented to what is happening around them that they are constantly on guard and unable to assess accurately whether something is a threat to them.

Using This Knowledge As a Caregiver

As the caregiver for a child with some the challenging behaviors listed above, it's not as important that you are able to analyze what the behavior means internally for your child, but that you understand that there are physiological reasons for those behaviors. There are professionals trained in seeing specific behaviors as a window into auditory and vestibular function, and in the next chapter we'll discuss what to look for and how to find one. But as a caregiver, being able to approach a child as a partner can make a huge difference. Taking a step back and looking at behavior through a different lens can have a great impact on what we decide to do about a child's behavior.

Instead of asking, "why is he doing this?" or "how can I make her stop doing this?" the better questions might be "What is making it so difficult for him to adapt in this situation?" and "what does this behavior provide for her, and can we get her that missing information?" When a child's behaviors are approached this way, we can provide the input and neurological skills so that the child can answer the question, "Is this new thing safe?" When a child can answer that question for themselves, their sense of exploration grows, their ability to learn about the world around them develops, and they begin to calmly and curiously navigate the world for themselves.

9 Making a Database About Your Child

Because the brain (especially mine) is prone to categorization, I have noticed that there are "types" of children. Each type exhibits fairly specific behaviors. During an evaluation, I may only see a child for a few minutes, but I can often guess some accurate things about their behavior outside the clinic. For example, if I begin an evaluation with a child and she is pulling a variety of toys from my shelves, but not really exploring any of them for more than a few seconds, I may turn to ask a parent, "Does she sleep well?" Many times the answer will be, "No! She's always been a terrible sleeper. How did you know?"

I have a method of categorizing children within the clinic that helps me narrow down where we might want to start with therapy, what kind of progress I can expect and what to recommend to a family. My system is definitely not bullet-proof. Children come in all shapes and sizes, with all kinds of home environments that can influence their behavior for better or worse. Behavior is a complex beast. But having an educated guess about the type of kiddo I might be dealing with saves me some time in the trial-and-error process. I'm going to share my categorization system here with you, and perhaps it will shed light on the type of child you might have in your life and how best to seek help for him or her. Be aware that these categories are absolutely NOT medical diagnoses. They represent more of a short-hand for me to think about what a child might be missing and what I can do for them as a therapist.

Sometimes the connection between a behavior and a possible dysfunction is obvious. A simple example is that of a child who is hypersensitive to auditory input. That child is likely to cover her ears often, become upset in noisy surroundings, and prefer the company of adults to children (because adults are naturally quieter).

If a child exhibits several of these behaviors, it might be safe to assume they have auditory hypersensitivity. Therapeutically, the next level of evaluation is to try to understand *the mechanism* of the hypersensitivity. Is the child hyper-responsive because she is unable to assess the direction from which a sound is coming, and therefore finds sounds more threatening (in which case she might exhibit a lot of anxiety)? Or is her tensor tympani muscle not activating to protect her hearing against loud noises (which is more likely to lead to discomfort and tantrums)? Specific behaviors she might exhibit could help us to answer these questions, then prescribe the appropriate intervention. It can be a very complex process and is by no means an exact science. Remember, people are complex systems and children are just little people.

In my classification system, there are two categories of auditory issues that can impact function: One category encompasses **auditory defensiveness and hypersensitivity**, which are grouped together because they both involve difficulties of the ear muscles in properly attenuating to different volumes and frequencies. The other category is **auditory hyposensitivity and/or processing problems,** both of which can involve hearing acuity and processing speed.

Correlatively, there are two categories of vestibular function; children may be either **vestibularly *hypo*sensitive** (not adequately registering or accurately sensing vestibular information) or **vestibularly *hyper*sensitive** (overreacting to vestibular input). While these gross generalizations are sometimes accurate, I find that there are some children who can vacillate between the extremes given their arousal level and the nature of the activity. There are even some children who only register vestibular input as an interesting sensation, but don't appear to incorporate it into their overall scheme when moving through the world.

For ease of understanding, vestibular dysfunction is divided into *hypo*sensitivity (not reactive enough) and *hyper*sensitivity (overly-reactive). Equally as important, however, may be the sensory system a child's brain primarily uses to "fill in" the information missing from their vestibular system. Do they depend excessively on visual input or proprioceptive input? The type of compensatory sensory information their brain prefers will greatly affect their overall presentation and behavior. This is one reason the reaction of the child to vestibular input during activities can vary greatly.

To further complicate things, most children have *both* auditory and vestibular issues. You may remember from the beginning of this book my mentioning that the auditory and vestibular systems are really the same system, sharing common anatomy and function, both being designed to sense movement. As a result, a child rarely has a difficulty with only one of these systems. However, it has been my experience that most developmentally-delayed children will have their function more greatly impacted either by vestibular disruptions or by auditory disruptions. Not as often will the problem be both, equally. These systems share anatomical structures and are part of complex physiological feedback loops that provide information to many parts of the brain and body simultaneously. Therefore, it is impossible to definitively point to a specific area of the cochlea, the vestibulum, or their respective neurological connections and say, "Aha! There's our culprit!"

In categorizing children and their behavior, my goal is to help you understand what type of child you have on your hands, and to give you a direction in which to seek help. Please pardon the cookbook approach taken here; this information is being simplified to make it easier to digest. Children are complicated. People are complicated. Please consider this to be one more lens through which you can view your child, to get a better understanding of their whole picture.

To sum up, dysfunction of the auditory system and the vestibular system can be rudimentarily divided into four categories based on which system is primarily involved, and whether that system is *hypo*sensitive, and therefore not providing accurate information, or *hyper*sensitive, and therefore creating a stronger reaction for a person than is necessary. This gives us four different categories of children who may be having difficulties:

- The Vestibularly-Hyposensitive Child
- The Vestibularly-Hypersensitivity Child
- The Auditorily-Hyposensitive Child
- The Auditorily-Hypersensitive Child

In my clinical practice, if I have correctly categorized a child with whom I am working, I can begin to predict what a parent will tell me about their preferences and behaviors. The predictive quality of these loose categories leads me to believe they have some merit. They give us a starting point to begin to discuss differences between children and the difficulties they may be having.

The Vestibularly-Hyposensitive Child

Confusingly, the vestibularly-*hypo*sensitive child usually presents as *hyper*active. They are typically disorganized in thought and behavior, and unlikely to enjoy sitting to play a game with another person. These children seem to be in constant motion, always more interested in the toy across the room than the one in front of them. They may have trouble with fine motor skills, perhaps because they haven't be able to devote sufficient attention to the smaller parts of their body. Or perhaps they simply don't feel comfortable sitting long enough to begin to master fine motor skills. Their lack of body-in-space awareness or knowledge of force interactions often translates to unintentionally aggressive behavior on the playground or excessive emotional stress when interacting with other children; they are often frustrated by their lack of understanding of the "rules" of cooperative play. It can be difficult to get them to participate in an activity that involves *trying* to keep their balance, because they seem to enjoy falling or crashing. Words that are commonly used to describe the vestibularly-hyposensitive child are words like "rambunctious", "impulsive", "disorganized" and "goofy." Older children tend to be the "class clowns." In each of the behavioral headings listed below, I have found certain tendencies and behaviors to be fairly common among children who don't receive strong enough or accurate enough information from their vestibular system.

Daily Bodily Functions: Younger children often have trouble sensing bowel and bladder needs, and are perhaps delayed in toilet-training. Sleep and the lack of it are long-standing problems for the child and their family. This child has trouble getting to sleep; often playing until late at night and then "passing out" wherever they are—but this can vary given how structured the home environment is. Regardless, this child usually appears to need a minimal amount of sleep, going to sleep late and often being the first one out of bed in the morning. When sleep does come it is hard and deep; it is difficult to wake this child.

Mobility: Early-walkers and babies who skip the crawling stage of mobility-development may be part of this group. While early walking might indicate a higher-than-normal level of coordination, they might trip over objects often, or have difficulty standing still. Older children will have trouble balancing on one foot or learning to skip. They may walk on their toes, seeking extra muscle input to compensate for lack of balance awareness. They may not be able to sit for meals. In fact they may rarely be caught sitting without a screen in front of them. Even to play with toys on the floor, they prefer to stand or squat, as opposed to sitting, needing input through their legs to feel grounded.

Ocular-Motor function: These children are likely to have difficulty maintaining a stable gaze, especially close-up, and therefore may be late or very inefficient readers. Eye-contact with others may be particularly challenging for them and the resulting disconnection with others can lead to a lack of empathy and understanding of others' emotional state.

Play and overall behaviors: Often, a parent's most pressing issue when dealing with a vestibularly-hyposensitive child is frequent, sudden and intense tantrums. Changes in routine or variation from what the child expects (being asked to stop what they are doing or another child getting in their way) results in a hyper-emotional tantrum. This may be related to their inability to form motor plans easily, because they don't innately understand why things happen when they do. They don't have a consistent relationship with gravity that allows them to predict and plan their motor movements with ease. So, when the motor plan they had in mind can't happen for whatever reason, it's very difficult for them to go with the flow and create a new plan.

More About Toe-Walking

<u>Toe-walking</u> is not in itself an indicator that a child is vestibularly-hyposensitive. Some children are so vestibularly-*hyper*sensitive that their brains stop using the vestibular system for information altogether. They are also likely to toe-walk. There are other ways to discriminate between the two categories, which will be reviewed in the section on vestibularly-hypersensitive children.

They are likely to nibble and snack throughout the day, both because they have trouble sitting for meals, and because they feel more grounded when there is additional feedback in the midline of their bodies, such as the feel of food in their mouths. This desire for stimulation along the midline of the body can lead to some annoying or weird behaviors. Most common is incessantly chewing on hair, shirt sleeves and collars, or toys, but some kids stimulate their midline by twirling their bangs, picking their nose, or especially in the case of boys, putting their hand down their pants.

Sitting to play with toys is a challenge and they tend to lose interest quickly in simple or quiet toys like puzzles or books. For this reason, they may be drawn to younger children, who tend to like more active play. Active play is usually their first choice, but when they become tired and need to rest, TV and video games can become an obsession; as though they cannot possibly sit still without a screen in front of them. In school, the need to bear weight through their legs to stay oriented can land them in hot water with the teacher for not staying seated. Most unique to this type of child is the tendency to try to execute unworkable plans of action: to stack things that aren't stackable or create rules to a game that are physically impossible. Because they don't know how a given plan of action will turn out, they execute many of the ideas that come to them, regardless of safety or propriety.

The Vestibularly-Hypersensitive Child

The vestibularly-hypersensitive child may also seek additional information through vision or proprioception. But they display some distinguishing characteristic that separate them from the vestibularly-hyposensitive group. These children often appear disconnected from the world around them; not engaging socially or not participating with the appropriate level of energy. This type of child is likely to be, but is not always, more sedentary. They may have age-appropriate (or better) fine motor skills, perhaps because sitting and working quietly is what they prefer to do. They may choose imaginative play over other types of play because it involves the least interaction with the concrete, physical environment.

They may have better-than-average verbal skills, perhaps because it helps them control their environment better to ask very specifically for what they want. These high verbal skills don't always translate into better communication or interpersonal connection, as these children seem *less* emotionally connected to others. They like to place things precisely during play and don't want items moved, and so they usually do not want to share their toys. Their emotional reactions to situations in which they are not in control can range from anxiety to anger. They may become upset when the routine is varied and may have less-frequent, but very intense and very long tantrums. They are likely to have low muscle tone throughout their body. If we look at the same category breakdown as we did for vestibularly-hyposensitve children, the vestibular over-reactor has behaviors that look different in many respects.

Daily Bodily Functions: Unlike hypo-sensitive children who have trouble falling asleep, these children often have trouble *staying* asleep, waking often during the night. If they struggle to get back to sleep, they may prefer having someone to sleep in the bed with them to anchor them and make them feel secure enough to return to sleep. Sometimes parents report that a child seems perfectly comfortable going to sleep in their own bed, but sneaks into mom and dad's bed during the night. Sometimes a child will express anxiety at bedtime because they anticipate awaking during the night and being disoriented; a night-light can often help.

Mobility: These children may crawl for a longer than others, being late walkers; in more severe cases, they may scoot on their bottom exclusively before transitioning to walking. They may be delayed in learning to navigate stairs because of a fear of heights or difficulty climbing. If they depend on proprioceptive input to stabilize themselves, they may respond poorly to new shoes or places where the walking surfaces change often. When seated, they lean excessively on their arms or surfaces or W-sit (see Fig. 9-1 on next page) during floor play, seeking a wide base of support and leaning on solid surfaces excessively. W-sitting can lead to very tight hip rotators as a child ages, making cross-legged sitting uncomfortable.

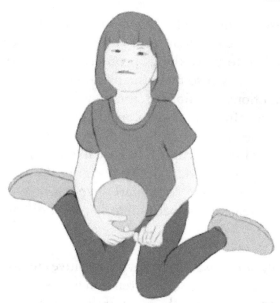

Fig. 9-1: Child in W-sitting posture

Ocular-motor function: Those children who are visually-dependent are likely to have difficulty tolerating rotary motion or become car-sick easily. They may have trouble locating objects because they have trouble moving their eyes with accuracy around a room. Proprioceptive seekers become goofier and more discombobulated as their eyes move around a space, such as when playing physical games with other children. Vestibularly-hypersensitive children are more likely to be early readers because they like stationary activities. Their ocular-motor function is better when stationary, and they may want neck or head support to read, propping their head up with their hand at a desk or lying in bed.

Play and Overall Behaviors: These children usually have low muscle tone, and may possibly have hyper-mobile joints. Instead of jumping in to trying new experiences, they may have an irrational or excessively fearful reaction to unfamiliar motion. Because they like more sedentary play with few surprises, they may choose to play alone or in clearly defined space, like a sandbox or closet, or play with friends who are older, or prefer the company of adults. Mostly, vestibularly-hypersensitive children like things to be "just so", so items can be easily located and the unexpected is minimized. They are likely to keep items in specific places, and may become upset when other children or adults move objects with which they are interacting, such as puzzle pieces. In very young children, a toy in front of them can sometimes be swapped with a different toy with very little reaction—as though pursuing the toy that was removed is too much work and the one they've just been given will do; therefore they appear easily content.

When vestibular sensations are too intense for a child with hypersensitivity, their brain may respond by "shutting off" that form of input. In this case, a vestibularly-*hyper*sensitive child and *hypo*sensitive one can look very much the same; clumsy, hyperactive, disoriented. So how can we tell what the essential problem is for a given child with these behaviors? I regard several indicators that help me find the right category when observing a child.

- Coordination: On the whole, a vestibularly-hyposensitive child will be more coordinated on the move than when they are stationary. Their skills tend to fall apart when seated. The hypersensitive child, however, may have good fine motor skills, but become discombobulated and clumsy when moving around the environment.

- Muscle tone: Vestibularly-hypersensitive children tend to have lower muscle tone. Because they prefer to have surfaces supporting them to maintain stability, they tend to lean into surfaces or their own limbs to stabilize themselves. This can lead to hyper-mobile joints, as they lean on their arms in full-extension, or limit the range of motion in their hips as they are given to W-sitting or wrapping their legs around the legs of a chair. Vestibularly-*hypo*sensitive children tend to have tightly-wound muscles, and lean on surfaces less; they are wiggle-worms when seated.

Vestibular therapy progress may be related to the sensitivity of a child's vestibular system, but is also influenced by how the child compensates for the missing information. Vestibularly-limited children sometimes need very large or very intense movements to trigger an awareness of vestibular input. The neural pruning that may have occurred because a child's vestibular input was not reliable needs to be overcome, and new neural connections need to

Breaking Through

When assessing a child's vestibular function, the rotating platform that is part of the Astronaut Training program is one of my favorite tools, because it provides information that I might not be able to obtain any other way. This platform is a two-foot by three-foot padded, rotating surface, on which I might have a child sit or lay down on to rotate them without their physical participation. I have a child sit on the board and I rotate them 10 times in one direction at a certain pace. I am looking for nystagmus; the eye-twitching movements that tell me the vestibular system is communicating with the ocular-motor muscles. If it is not present or is limited, then the conclusion may be that I am dealing with a child who may be vestibularly-hyposensitive.

However, I sometimes find that, when a child who initially appears vestibularly-hyposensitive lies on their side on the board and I rotate them 10 times, when I stop they have a *hyper*sensitive response. Their eyes open wide, and they roll onto their bellies and grip the ground with fear and anxiety. The intense and very different movement of rotating the head in the vertical plane, in a sense, *broke through* their resistance to taking in vestibular input, which is good; but the sensations were so unusual for them, they didn't know how to process them. My job as the OT is to wake up their vestibular system, then provide the right kind of movement to help them begin to process vestibular sensations as part of how they move through the world all day, every day.

be made. This might involve taking away the sense that they have been depending on to compensate for the lack of vestibular input.

If I've seen evidence in the clinic that they are the type of child who uses their vision and visually locks onto objects to stay oriented, then I might have them swing in my net swing. The net swing is wrapped around them (think of a fish in a net), so they are safe from falling, no matter how large the arc of the swing or how erratic. This is useful if I need to provide the child with very large movements for sensations to register. The net also provides a visual barrier; they can see through the net, but it's harder for their eyes to lock onto a specific object to anchor themselves as the swing moves. It's like trying to watch a ball game through a chain-link fence, you can follow the action, but it's harder to lock onto specifics.

If I believe the child is a proprioception seeker, I will try to limit their access to proprioception while moving, such as rotating them on the rotary board, or swinging on a platform swing. The surface really doesn't give them much information about their movement because it feels the same whether they are moving or still. My particular treatment approach is outlined more in-depth in Appendix A. Your child's therapist may take a different approach to vestibular treatment, but they should be able to articulate why they chose a movement or activity for your child and what they hope to gain.

The Auditorily-Hyposensitive Child

I find that generally, children with auditory hyposensitivity and/or auditory processing problems are more likely to have a complex medical history. This may include premature birth, a history of ear infections, severe allergies and/or tonsil and adenoid difficulties, or prolonged hospitalization. With prematurity, the *in utero* practice of listening to bone-conducted sound gets cut short and development of auditory foreground and background is interrupted. In the case of ear infections, allergies, and tonsil and adenoid enlargement, variable sound sensitivity to environmental noises from day-to-day make auditory input unreliable as a source of information for the child. Neural pruning eliminates some of the neural pathways for that unreliable information; connections that should have been made stronger if the information had been consistent. For children who spent extended time in the hospital after birth, it is possible that their auditory sense became overwhelmed in such a noisy environment (with beeping machines and constant communication of others) and may have selectively shut down as a method of self-preservation. These are all, of course, suppositions.

Daily Bodily Functions: Because listening is the first truly bilateral function of the body and brain, sensory changes that prevent hearing correctly through both ears may create difficulty for a child in developing a sense of where the middle of their body is. As a result, they may lack orientation to the different parts of their body because they lack a definitive "center" on which to orient a schematic of themselves. This especially applies to the muscles of the face, where decreased body awareness is compounded by a lack of visual confirmation of movement. Low body awareness might also mean a delay in potty-training. They may have a hard time orienting themselves securely on furniture and play equipment, and be surprised by sensations (usually unpleasantly so).

Mobility: These children may often run into doors or corners, bang their head on surfaces, and seem unaware of the size of their space, because their ability to use echolocation is impaired. This lack of awareness of surrounding space sometimes results in delayed attainment of mobility milestones, like crawling and walking. Sometimes, motor milestones are initiated by an attempt to get to an object just out of reach; since our depth perception begins as an auditory function. These children may not be able to orient to things that are *just outside* their reach that should motivate them become mobile.

Ocular-motor function: Decreased awareness of the precise point in space from which a sound is coming can decrease a child's drive to complete the hearing-moving-looking triad, resulting in trouble directing their eyes with accuracy. They may often struggle to find desired objects, even if they are in plain sight, resulting in frustration. They may choose to keep their eyes on a toy or object in front of them instead of making eye contact when spoken to, decreasing opportunities for social connection. And ocular-motor difficulties understandably affect reading ability, because their eyes have trouble making small movements across a page.

Play and Overall Behaviors: Speech difficulties are common, ranging from minor articulation errors to completely unintelligible speech. Verbal children may still exhibit a constricted emotional range, both in their speech and facial expression, or have overly-concrete thinking, a lack of sense of humor or inability to comprehend idioms. They may miss social cues and misunderstand social situations. For example, many of these children are confused by the concept that someone laughing because they did something cute or funny is different from someone "laughing at them." At times, these children are surprised by other's behaviors; for example, when mom finally loses her temper over a child's repeated misbehavior. The child may have missed the warning tone in mom's voice as she asked him to stop a behavior several times. When she becomes upset or punishes the child, he is truly surprised.

Because they aren't as comfortable with verbal communication, in play they are likely to choose playground activities over imaginative play with others, choose games and activities below their age-level, or act immaturely. An impaired ability to trust the auditory sense as an early-warning system can lead these children to be easily visually distracted and they may have a hard time maintaining focus on a chosen task. As they age, academics can become challenging as they struggle with reading and spelling. Not hearing the very subtle differences in the sounds of letters (most specifically vowels) results in an inability to sound out words and can lead to frustration with academic tasks. These children may also have difficulty remembering lessons from day-to-day; both because they don't perceive the emotional content of others' speech does not convey to them, allowing them to make concrete memories, and because they lack an orientation in time from moment to moment.

The Auditorily-Hypersensitive Child

In more impaired cases of auditory-hypersensitivity, the tensor tympani muscle is not protecting the ear from louder sounds and a child's brain might respond by shutting down attention to *all* incoming auditory information. Or a child might only have a persistent startle reflex or cover their ears often. Because the level of impairment and the reaction can create different behaviors, it is hard to create a picture of a "typical" auditorily-hypersensitve child. In mild cases of auditory defensiveness and hypersensitivity, a child may be fairly capable in most situations, with minimal motor-skills deficits and fair-to-good communication skills. They may only have sensitivity to certain pitches, or be unable to tolerate parties or crowds. Other behaviors for auditorily-hypersensitive children are directly related to their sense of hearing: covering their ears, or having a strong reaction to specific sounds that other people can tolerate. Some behaviors may seem more related to personality and preferences: negative reaction to or avoidance of certain people without reason (which could be due to sensitivity to their vocal pitch), limited vocal inflection and/or monotone voice, a fear of dogs or balloons, or trouble using public bathrooms, because of the odd acoustics and loud noises.

In cases of extreme auditory hypersensitivity, the child's behaviors can be a bit harder to analyze. These children tend to have very robust tantrums. Some appear auditorily-*hypo*sensitive because they have stopped responding to *any* auditory cues. These children are likely to have limited communication skills (they may be non-verbal) and may make frequent, meaningless vocalizations to block incoming sound. I believe this was the case with my friend Brandon from the introduction to this book.

Daily Bodily Functions: These children often seem to have minimal sleep requirements and they may have a strong preference to sleep only when a trusted person is in the room. The difference between these children and vestibularly-challenged children, who also need company to sleep, is that these kids don't necessarily have to be in physical contact with someone else; having them in the room is usually enough. They can suffer from large swings in alertness level, from withdrawn and lethargic when made to listen as *the* activity (such as in class), to hyperactive and upset very quickly (such as when surrounded by overwhelming noise, like in the school cafeteria).

Mobility: While they are likely to be on-schedule in meeting motor milestones like crawling and walking, they may not seem to have a desire to continue to explore their environment. They are not likely to wander off. Although they may seem disconnected, they want to stick to trusted person or familiar location.

Ocular-motor function: Because of the potential for impaired sound-localization skills, they may have trouble visually scanning their environment during play. This can limit their preferred activities to near-play with small toys or TV and video games in which the eyes don't travel much. Playground play might be uncomfortable for them if they struggle with visually pursuing objects, like other children running by.

Play and Overall Behaviors: Their avoidance of playground situations might result in their choice to play alone or with one or two trusted friends. They may have a history of biting other children, especially when younger. Biting could be a result of being unpleasantly surprised by another child's proximity; they didn't hear that child approach or wasn't aware of them, then they are suddenly startled and need to say, "get away from me!" When the child enters their space or moves an object near them, biting could be a defensive response, even if their "victim" didn't touch them or wasn't trying to interact with them. The quieter company of adults or older children may be their choice and they may avoid or react negatively to younger children, whose noises and movements are less predictable. This can be a struggle for families in which the child has younger siblings; creating a lot of fights between the children in which refereeing is required. And of course, there is often the most noticeable hallmark of a hypersensitive child: they cover ears often and display fear of balloons, automatic-flush toilets, dogs, and other things that make unexpected noises.

Connecting the behaviors listed above with the potential auditory reasons for them requires quite a few leaps of faith. The connection between sensory input to the child and resulting behavioral or motor output may not be obvious, and requires some imagination to put oneself in the child's auditory shoes. But after having treated so many children who struggle with auditory hyposensitivity and processing problems, and seeing behaviors and motor skills improve without "teaching" the child anything related to those skills and behaviors, I do believe that many difficulties for neurodiverse children stem from auditory issues. Several behaviors, to varying degrees, are common to most children with auditory hyposensitivity, strengthening my own conclusions about which children can benefit from auditory therapy.

Does Your Child Need Therapy?

When trying to help a child make their lives easier and more comfortable, we have to list the things that can be wrong with a child. I find "wrong" to be a useful, but sometimes damaging, word. It's important to stress that being different does not always mean something is wrong and needs to be corrected. Let's visit the idea first that not all children who are different need therapy. Some kids are challenging, some kids are quirky. Most quirky kids benefit greatly from an adult in their lives who understands that some things are challenging for them, and that's ok. Having that understanding adult might be enough to help them overcome challenges during childhood. If your child is succeeding in many aspects of life, but is just a "little weird" about some things, that might be ok. Perhaps just implementing a few suggestions and adapting your child's daily routine or environment will be enough to help your child overcome difficulties and feel better and safer. However, if your child is having problems that are creating a sense of failure at life (either for them or for you), then it might be time to seek the help of a professional.

Parents in my clinic and casual parenting acquaintances will tell me about their child and ask me, "What do you think? Should my child be getting therapy?" My answer to this is always, "Is the problem your child having impairing his or her ability to participate in life in a way that is acceptable to you? Is the problem your child is having impairing your function as a family?" Keep in mind that these thresholds for "participation" and "function" are different for every family. When posed with this question, I've had several families forego therapy for their children. The time and effort commitment was too great in relation to the benefit for a child or family that was already fairly functional. Two of these instances come to mind in which, had I been the parent in the situation, I would have had my child in therapy because their particular issues would have been real problems in my household. One child would not sleep in her room through the night at seven years of age, and the other nine-year-old child would not eat any food that hadn't been prepared to exact specifications by his mother, so she toted around a cooler of food for him. In my family, these issues would have impaired our ability to function as a family, but these mothers did not feel the accommodations they made for their child were overwhelming. Each family must assess the value of what they expect to gain in therapy, then decide whether to dedicate the effort and expense.

For almost every one of us, a perceived weakness is also a strength. For example, I am a pretty blunt person. Sometimes I lack tact or say things too forcefully, and I hurt people's feelings. But my honesty is valued by people closest to me, as they can always trust that I say what I mean, and I mean what I say. This is the same dynamic for many of the quirks that make daily life difficult for some children. I don't personally know Temple Grandin, the animal scientist, autism activist and author, but after reading her writing, I think that if I had a magic wand and told her that I could wave that wand and eliminate her autism, she wouldn't take me up on my offer. She highly values the associational and visual thinking that is a result of her autism. It has allowed her to design amazing animal-handling equipment that has positively impacted the lives of hundreds of thousands of animals. But, if I offered a way in which she could better express herself, more easily connect with those she loved and better understand the social constructs of the world that confound her, she might take me up on *that* offer.

Good and proper therapy should be a little like that magic wand. It should create more ease for a child in connecting with others and being more adaptable. It certainly should not continually frustrate them by asking them to have skills that are impossible for them without the underlying neurological connections. After reading this book, you may have decided that this approach to therapy would be a good step for your child. Perhaps you would like to learn more about auditory therapy, in which case I would refer you to Dorinne Davis's book, *The Cycle of Sound* (see References). But, perhaps instead, you would like to try some small interventions or changes based on what your child needs. While that's not the focus of this book, there are other books out there with wonderful suggestions for adapting your child's environment to optimize their function. My favorites include *Raising a Sensory-Smart Child* by Lindsey Biel and Nancy Peske and *Sensational Kids* by Lucy Jane Miller (also in References).

Perhaps appropriate therapy is not geographically available to you, or you'd like to limit the number of appointments your child has outside the home. You could set out to gather more information, become trained in some forms of therapy yourself, or purchase a system that is commercially available (more about that in the next chapter).

For very involved and complex children, there is sometimes no substitute for a knowledgeable therapist engaged in an effective give-and-take relationship with a child; a therapist that observes the child's responses and changes in every session and understands how to interpret those responses therapeutically, to guide effective treatment. If you have found one of these dynamic therapists, keep her number! The situations in which having a professional intervene to help your child could be:

- Your child's impairments are so severe that you don't know where to begin.

- You prefer to be your child's supportive caregiver and cheerleader, and to leave the task of challenging your child in uncomfortable ways to a professional.

- You may be unsure of technical aspects of treatment and would like to have professional guidance.

- You may need access to special equipment that is available in a well-outfitted clinic.

After careful consideration, and perhaps an evaluation by a professional, you have decided that your time, energy, and money would best benefit your child by finding them appropriate auditory and vestibular therapy. What does that look like? As a lay-person, you might want some definitive hallmarks, which I'll give you in the next chapter. But also important when selecting a therapist, are the following questions to consider:

- What is this person's experience with children like mine?

- Does this person seem competent? Are they able to answer my questions knowledgably? (note: it should not be off-putting to a therapist that you did some research before seeing them and have specific questions. Similarly, it should not be insulting to them if you research the information they provide to you more in-depth.)

- Does my child like coming to therapy? This one can be a bit tricky. If your child is one who does not like challenges or new situations, then it may take longer for your child to reach their comfort level. But reach it, they should. And if it takes more than one month, it might be time to start asking questions.

- If your child is already receiving therapy, ask yourself if you can point to at least three concrete, positive changes in your child since they began therapy. Not three things the therapist has told you they are working on, but three behaviors you *know* are better than they were before therapy.

If you know you are looking for a therapist who considers the auditory and vestibular systems paramount in treatment, there are some specific things to look for in their clinic or workspace, and in their approach. In the next chapter, we'll explore exactly what to look for.

10   **Signposts**

At seven-years-old, Sean's quick wit and, to my great pleasure, love of movies and 80s music, was evident from the start. His kind heart was often overshadowed by strong tantrums, severe sensory reactions to certain foods, physical fighting with others in school, and hyper-emotional reactions to being corrected. After two months of treatment, he was able to adjust so much better to new routines and unfamiliar foods, that the family was able to take their first *enjoyable* family vacation ever. His mother was thrilled that he wasn't overwhelmed by the crash of ocean waves or the feel of the sand, and that the change in schedule didn't cause him to melt down, as it had on previous vacations. "Robin, it was so wonderful to have a fun family vacation. They've never really been fun before," she admitted, her eyes a bit teary.

One day, at the end of Sean's session, his mom asked me, "Robin, what's your opinion of ABA therapy? Do you think we should keep going?" I knew Sean had been in ABA (Applied Behavioral Analysis) for two years and was continuing to go, because it had been suggested by his doctor. "Why do you ask?" I wondered aloud. His mother told me that Sean's father was surprised by Sean's remarkable progress in only two months of our time together. His father was frustrated because the professionals they had trusted didn't seem to know that this "therapy accelerator" was available. None of them had suggested this approach, with which Sean seemed to be advancing more quickly than ever before.

I completely understood. I felt the same frustration every time I began to work with a child who had been in therapy for quite some time, making only small gains. While I can't make estimations for children receiving speech and physical therapy, it has been my experience that only children who are non-verbal, have compounding neurological difficulties (like a stroke or cerebral palsy) or have extreme and destructive behaviors need occupational therapy for more than six months. For families continuing to take time out of their schedules to bring their child to therapy after six months, I would hope that the pay-off is significant, such as sleeping through the night, uttering a first word and continuing to build vocabulary, or being able to integrate into a classroom setting.

But how can a parent stop taking their child to therapy if that child hasn't met her goals yet? If she's still not a functional, healthy member of her family and community, why would a parent stop doing the only things recommended by professionals? Parents still might not know where to turn or what to do next. Five-year-old Liam's mom, Ashley, had a degree in early childhood education. She knew something was not right in Liam's speech development from a young age, and took him to see an audiologist, who did indeed diagnose him with auditory processing problems. But, she became quite frustrated when he didn't qualify for speech services, because his verbal communication scored within acceptable ranges when tested. "Robin," said an exasperated Ashley, "there was so much else wrong with him—his attention, his lack of *real* understanding— but no one told me those problems were related to his listening. No one told me there was a therapy for what was wrong with him. If we hadn't met you, how would we have found out what could help him?" Ashley described the frustrating dead-end that some parents run into in trying to seek help for their child. The "right" answers are out there, but it feels like dumb luck when a family finds them.

Throughout this book, we've reviewed how a functional vestibular and auditory system can inform other sensory systems for normal development. And we've touched on what can go wrong and what that might look like in a child's development. Understanding how your child might be wired differently can help you help them cope with their world from day-to-day. But all of us, as parents, therapists and educators, would like for the children we love to do more than just cope, but to navigate their world as independently and happily as possible. It *is* possible to give a child specific sensory input that helps their brain establish the right connections, to understand and participate in their world more smoothly and confidently, but it has to be the correct type of input to address the neurological needs of the child. That's when effective treatment with

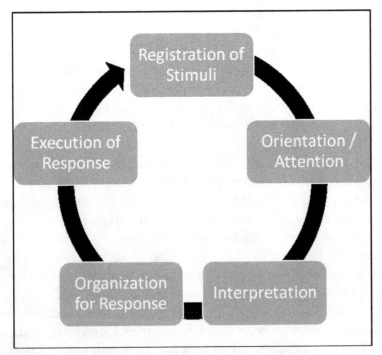

Fig. 10-1: Cycle of functional response to stimuli.

the appropriate methods can make huge differences for children and their families.

The illustration in Fig. 10-1 from Williamson and Anzalone's (2001) *Sensory Integration and Self-Regulation in Infants and Toddlers* elegantly illustrates the normal cycle that must take place during a child's *appropriate* responses to the environment and his learning of new information. The actions of the vestibular and auditory systems are crucial to every step in the cyclical nature of responding to stimuli.

One must first register the stimulus. If it is auditory, a child must be able to register it through functional ear mechanisms and also recognize it as novel within the environment. He must orient to the location of the sound; this involves knowing where he is in the space of the environment (a vestibular function) and locating the sound in space (an auditory function). His brain must send this information to the correct part of the brain and make a sensory match, or mismatch, to tell him what his next physical or mental response should be. He must organize his body for a response; to ignore and filter the stimulus out, or turn and look for more information, allowing his vestibular system and his auditory system to feed information to his body and brain about how he is moving in space, how he is moving around his core, and how the environment should shift auditorily and visually because of that movement. He must have the motor coordination for an effective response; his eyes must travel to an accurate point in space for sound localization, his head must turn with accurate control around his middle to stabilize his eyes. And on and on.

The seemingly-simple act of responding to the ringing of a doorbell is actually very physically and neurologically complex. In treatment, it's important to address the point at which this complicated chain of events has broken down. Many forms of therapy present the same stimulus repeatedly, then tell the child what response is expected. Asking for a motor or behavioral response, such as visual attention to a stimulus the adult has deemed important, can make very little sense to the child. They might be able to force themselves to look at an object or person, but they won't understand *why*. It's a bit like asking a fourth-grader to write a 20-page essay on astrophysics. Does a typical fourth-grader know how to write? Yes. But there are years of sensory input, cognitive development and education required before the child has the skills to complete such a complex assignment. Asking for a product when the child doesn't have the necessary neurological foundation, skills, and information can be frustrating for everyone involved, even when that task is broken down into its component parts and practiced. Yet this is a common approach in most therapies.

A child may have the capacity to learn by rote the appropriate response to a question or situation. But unless the proper functional response is their *natural* chain of events, it will always be harder for them to react and adapt to their changing environment than it should be. Being able to adapt and respond effectively to one's environment is the *definition of function*, and we all want our children to be as functional and independent as possible in every developmental stage.

With the auditory and vestibular systems being the pillars on which further development rest, difficulties in either or both can lead to developmental delays specific to where the dysfunction arises. Careful observation of a child's behaviors and reactions to sensations can indicate to another person which of these systems might not be providing accurate or complete information, so that we might be able to provide sensory input that fills in those informational gaps. Without exception, there isn't a child that comes to my clinic that doesn't need some form of vestibular and/or auditory therapy. If those systems were functioning optimally, the child wouldn't have come to my clinic for treatment in the first place. Treatment may include other types of intervention; such as eating practice, puzzles and other fine motor practice, or sensory interventions, such as weighted blankets and therapeutic brushing. I think of these interventions as adjunct therapies to effective auditory and vestibular therapy.

Auditory therapy can come in various packages. They have names like Integrated Listening System, the Listening Program, Samonas, and Tomatis. All these programs are based on the same principles regarding how the human ear responds to sound. Each system involves hearing electronically-modified music and sounds through headphones. Some elements of programs vary, perhaps involving bone-conduction input through headphones, or having a component involving the child's participation using their own voice.

Older children often come to my clinic because they are having academic problems, particularly with reading or writing. In the case of reading difficulties, two different mechanisms might be at play. The child could be having difficulty moving her eyes across a page in a coordinated manner, or she could be having difficulty hearing individual speech sounds, making associating those sounds with visual representations (letters and words) more difficult.

If 9-year-old Janice is having trouble reading and I notice that her eyes do not team up well and she is afraid of climbing on my swing because she doesn't like when her feet leave the ground, I will know that spatially-enhanced sound will need to be part of her treatment program. Spatially-enhanced albums are recorded natural sounds engineered to be immersive, so that a sound coming through the headphones sounds as if it really is a bird in the trees above, or a fly buzzing in from the right. This will enhance Janice's ability to move her eyes around her environment with greater accuracy in response to sounds when she is *not* wearing the headphones, because she practiced this skill for an hour each day. If her eyes move with more accuracy and coordination, then moving them across a page to read will become easier. Because Janice also demonstrated gravitational insecurity (fear of movement when her feet left the ground) she may be having trouble hearing how far away the ground is once she is not in contact with it. Spatially-enhanced sound can positively affect this behavior as well (Frick and Young, p. 90).

Eleven-year-old Susan may also be having difficulty with reading, but it may be related to an inability to hear individual speech sounds. In this case, electronically-modulated instrumental music can be helpful in helping her to understand the difference in vowel sounds, as vowel sounds are in the same frequency range as some instruments. Consonant sounds, however, are sometimes in very high frequency ranges. These sounds are even difficult for adults to hear differences in, which is why we say "'D' as in 'dog' and 'B' as in 'boy'" when communicating letters to others. So Susan's programs would eventually include albums engineered to enhance the higher frequency ranges of speech; 2000 Hz and above.

Or perhaps the academic problems that are concerning teachers are related to poor writing. 12-year-old Tim cannot legibly write a complete sentence. His evaluation revealed poor vestibular function and motor coordination, while seated, for which he will need vestibular therapy. But his body awareness and bilateral coordination can also be greatly enhanced by music that emphasizes lower frequencies and strong rhythms, so these would also be included in his treatment program.

We All Use Music to Move Better

Researchers have found that parts of the brain, outside of neurological centers directly related to hearing, are also activated by rhythm and pitch differentials; particularly the areas dealing with visual-spatial processing, reaching and grasping tasks, and timing and sequencing of movements. This is why our movements become more coordinated and smoother when we put them to music, as in an aerobics class. We can use these features of instrumental music to enhance a child's ability to estimate where their pencil point must make contact with the paper and how to coordinate their movements to accomplish this.

Adjunct Therapies

As I realized how effective this form of therapy was, techniques I previously used to help children adapt to their environment, like social skills practice, or tactile and sensory desensitization (like the Wilbarger Sensory Therapeutic Brushing Protocol), or ocular-motor games and activities, served new roles in therapy. Those techniques were now used to reinforce emerging skills, moved later in the treatment sequence when a child was more neurologically ready, or used to measure gains in skills that auditory and vestibular improvements were uncovering.

I might continue to play ocular-motor skill games or have social-interaction-based sessions with my clients, but more and more often these activities were an opportunity for me to see how their abilities had developed as a result of treatment and to tell me which direction to continue in. They were no longer practice activities for skills we were *trying* to develop. As this therapy reconnected parts of the brain that had been short-circuited, a child already used these new connections in the course of their regular day: completing school work, playing with friends, participating in activities with their family. Many times, I no longer needed to *directly* address sleeplessness, or tactile sensitivity, or hyperactivity, or reading difficulties. With increasing frequency, the children I treated began to adapt to the challenges of their environment all by themselves. The situations in which a given child usually had difficulty simply became easier for them.

Some dysfunctional behaviors improved early on in treatment of the child's auditory system and vestibular system, but not always. Sometimes, I did need to continue with other treatment techniques; to increase a child's body awareness or directly address constant movement. But those interventions were so much more effective when combined with or completed after vestibular and auditory treatment. Some of the treatment techniques that I continue to find useful are listed in Appendix A.

Pleasant Surprises

There have been times in my professional life when my faith in this type of therapy was reinforced despite misgivings I had. Such was the case of Lisa, who had suffered a stroke at the age of two during a heart surgery, but didn't meet me in therapy until she was five-years-old. I wasn't sure if this approach would help. Was her stroke too far in the past? The stroke had left her with very tight neck muscles and limited range of motion for neck rotation, and one eye that didn't want to play along when she shifted her gaze. This created years of not being able to close the listening-moving-looking loop effectively. Hoping to enhance her use of this neurological loop and loosen her neck muscles, I began using spatially-recorded sound with her. And voila! Over the course of several weeks, her eyes aligned and her depth perception improved. This helped her to be more confident in her movements through space, relaxing her muscles and allowing for greater freedom of movement.

There have been situations in which a child's developmental "holes" filled in. Pre-schooler Alice had received OT as an infant, as part of the early intervention program, and her family's first experience with OT had not gone well. That therapist was confounded by her odd crawling style of keeping one leg out, with her foot flat on the floor. She tried to correct this by wrapping adult ankle-weights around Alice's leg to *make* her crawl like she should. It didn't work (of course) and her parents were unimpressed by OT in general, thinking it ineffective and a bit of torture for Alice. When Alice was three-years-old, they agreed to have her participate in therapy with me. Weirdly enough, as she made all kinds of other progress, her parents noticed that she was crawling on all-fours while playing. At three years old, she didn't need to crawl for mobility, as she could walk. But kids play on the floor, and now Alice was crawling during play, naturally, for the first time. We certainly hadn't been practicing this skill in the clinic. It just "magically" got better once her vestibular developmental "holes" were filled in.

Some children meet me after they fall outside the developmental "golden zone" of birth-to-five. Oliver's mother had found me online, through a presentation of mine that was posted, and she believed I could help her son. He was 13-years-old and had struggled in school his entire life. He had worked hard, played sports, and was a social kid, but academics remained something that brought him to tears. Could this approach really help a child as functional as Oliver? Would it be worth his parents' time? After a couple of months, it was obvious that Oliver found school easier and more enjoyable, and his grades had improved. But as a side-benefit, long-standing speech issues I didn't know he had, because they were so minimal, improved. His mom was so surprised to hear him say "specifically" and "spaghetti" correctly, after mispronouncing them for years.

These anecdotes are certainly not scientific proof of anything. But they surprised me, and are only a few of the surprises I have encountered in working with children doing this type of therapy. Those unexpected improvements, which I have come to call "collateral improvements" really aren't explainable any other way. These children improved in skills they weren't directly "practicing", had been in other forms of therapy in the past, and only now improved in these areas while participating in auditory and vestibular therapy. It may not be a randomized controlled trial, but it certainly gave me pause.

Caveats

Some version of vestibular therapy and auditory therapy outlined above should be available at your child's therapy center. However, there are some exceptions to this: hospital-based therapy will involve children who are more medically-fragile and may have restrictions on what is available and safe for their population, and school-based therapy is often restricted by budgetary concerns and the legal requirement for therapy to be directly related to the child's educational function. But in an outpatient clinic, I find the equipment and processes I've outlined here to be not just desirable, but necessary for effective, efficient treatment.

Early in therapy, I often have to quell some alarm in parents when it appears that their child is becoming *less* coordinated, getting banged up more on the playground or falling over more often. In my experience this is a brief period of adjustment as the child's brain attempts to understand this new input that it may have been ignoring for some time. I imagine it's somewhat like growing a third arm. It might take you a while to figure out how to use it, but after a period of adjustment, you'd be more efficient with every task in your day.

There have been several situations in which a child did not make the improvements that I expected at his or her initial evaluation, even after months of therapy. That said, each child did make *some* improvement; just not what as much as hoped. While some situations remain a mystery, there are a couple of categories of neurological differences or medical histories in children that I find do not respond as well to this therapy. They are:

- Children with a suspected or known history of exposure to alcohol or drugs *in utero*. Perhaps there is a level of neurological damage so early in the developmental process for these children that their responses to stimuli are more difficult to normalize.

- Children who have experienced significant trauma, especially before developing language skills. Possibly, these children are defensive against the orienting response this therapy is designed to elicit, perhaps because their memory of the trauma is not associated with the past. Because they were not able to process the memory using words and associate it as a story that *happened* to them, orienting to their bodies brings back the trauma as a flashback that *is happening* to them and detaching their awareness is a defense mechanism (van der Kolk, 2014).

- Older children (above 10 years old or so) who have limited speech and are self-injurious or physically aggressive. When older children participate in this therapy, there can be times during which it is uncomfortable. We are trying to change neural patterns that have ingrained themselves over years. For verbal children, we can usually talk through these difficulties. But for aggressive kids, therapy sometimes can only progress to the point at which they are simply physically more coordinated when they strike out, but the behavior itself doesn't change. The increase in physical skills created by their increased body awareness only serves to make it more difficult for caregivers. Caution is recommended with children with these types of difficulties.

Why Isn't Everyone Doing This?

If the effectiveness of this type of therapy is so obvious, why isn't every occupational, speech or physical therapist using it? That is an excellent question, and quite frankly it's the reason why I wrote this book. There are several potential reasons why vestibular and auditory therapy are not more frequently employed or are not more readily available. Foremost, a therapist must be exposed to the theories on which these treatment practices are founded. I wasn't introduced to these theories in school, and the feedback I receive after giving lectures to other therapists, educators and parents indicates to me that they weren't either.

In any professional therapy program, a student is learning anatomy and physiology, disease processes, and treatment techniques that apply to people all across the spectrum of life, from newborns to the elderly. There is a lot of information to convey in the short time students are in school. Professionals take classes and workshops in specific techniques in areas that interest them after they graduate. But choosing a workshop to attend is a bit like shooting in the dark, especially in geographically underserved areas, where a therapist might not be working with another professional with whom to share ideas and seek guidance.

The academic world stresses the use of "evidence-based practice." Students are instructed that there should be peer-reviewed evidence based on rigorous studies for the treatment techniques they employ. This presents quite a conundrum for those of us that work with people. People are complex systems, with changes to any aspect of a person's life having multiple possible results. Within the complex human body, the vestibular and auditory systems have myriad connections with multiple parts of the brain, as illustrated in previous chapters. So, creating a rigorous study in which changing one variable, such as vestibular experience, would have predictable results that could be outlined in an elegant hypothesis is all but impossible.

However, there have also been studies that investigate some aspects of vestibular treatment, particularly studies involving Sensory Integration (SI) treatment. These studies suffer from a lack of rigor and fidelity to just *one* model of SI treatment. "SI treatment" can be interpreted to mean something different in every study. This contributes to a rather inconclusive body of knowledge regarding SI treatment's effectiveness. Not only that, but SI treatment was originally designed to be a cooperative effort between the child and therapist to create and execute activities that coordinate various sensory inputs toward achieving a specific goal. That's very high-level stuff that requires a cooperative, communicative child. The children I meet for therapy are often so disconnected, frightened or impaired that they are not ready for this type of therapy. There exists no rigorous treatment protocol on which a therapist can depend when a child is too dysfunctional to participate in true SI therapy.

There are studies on both auditory and vestibular function being conducted in several different branches of the academic environment. But each of these specialties is looking at one small piece of the larger puzzle. This is the nature of academic research. The neurobiologist studies the part of the brain that helps us produce speech. The early childhood researcher documents how babies communicate and what that means in the context of development. Another researcher studies the nature of vestibular dysfunction at the chemical level. All of these studies can be pieces of the whole picture, but it takes quite a large step backward, further away from hard evidence to see how all these pieces fit together in the context of an actual child.

Even after a therapist has been exposed to the theories of auditory and vestibular therapy, they may choose not to use these forms of therapy. Why might this be? Well, it may be because they haven't experienced first-hand the tremendous and otherwise inexplicable changes I have seen in children in my clinic. But I have a personal theory that the therapy community is resistant to this approach is *because* it is so simple. If one has a master's or doctorate degree, one expects their job to be very complicated. Therefore, it must be somewhat labor-intensive, either cognitively or physically. But this type of treatment, especially in its initial phases, seems very passive, for both the child and the therapist. We are simply exposing a child to the auditory or vestibular input that will help to rewire their brain. They are *just* listening, or *just* being moved through space. We aren't asking them for a motor response or really much participation at all. That seems counterintuitive to most therapists.

Not only that, but many of the gains for the child are made *outside* the clinic. After a week of listening to a new album, I get the really fun opportunity to see what new things that child can do. Or, after I have helped a child tune in to vestibular input, they may not have made any gains in physical skills (and on occasion might even be *less* coordinated) as a result of the session. But then, they spend the next few days incorporating new sensations and information into the tasks they do every day. When they return to me, I again get to have fun seeing what new skills they are capable of. But, it's not me, as the therapist, that did anything for the child. I was just the tool to expose them to the stimulus they needed. Some therapists, I think, can't separate themselves from the process of therapy enough to accept that they are not the agent of change for the child.

I came to rely on auditory and vestibular treatment in my clinic, not through evidence-based practice, but through *practice-based evidence*. The evidence I saw was available in every treatment session; in the child who could stack seven blocks instead of two after swinging in the net swing. The child who did not notice my offered hand to hold at the beginning of a session, but could take my hand when I offered it while listening to an auditory therapy album. The child who was petrified of climbing up the rock wall, but after one week of listening to a specific album, was no longer afraid. The child who participates in three weeks of regimented vestibular therapy and begins to read more fluidly and willingly. These moments were the proof I was looking for that what I could provide would make a difference in the lives of children.

Bringing It All Together

When I provide treatment to address the child's auditory and vestibular deficits, the caregivers and I work as a team to gather information about how they are responding to the prescribed treatment. In her book *Sound Bodies Through Sound Therapy*, Dorinne Davis states that "when both the vestibular system and the cochlea are affected, it is important to work on the vestibular system. By stimulating the muscles of the middle ear first, auditory hypersensitivity is reduced and the vestibular system can be rebalanced" (p. 140). It has indeed been my experience that both auditory and vestibular treatment are usually necessary. I have been in several situations in which I was able to administer either auditory or vestibular treatment alone, perhaps because there was not auditory equipment available, or because a child could not tolerate much movement. In each case, the expected results were only partially achieved until the child was in a position to experience both forms of treatment.

With almost every child that has successfully overcome the dysfunction or behavior for which their family was seeking help, there have usually been additional behaviors or problems that also improved. Often, caregivers aren't expecting improvement in some areas as a result of OT because those areas are typically the domains of other treatment providers. For example, poor communication or speech articulation problems are usually the purview of speech therapists. The increase in sound sensitivity and/or speed of processing as a result of auditory therapy usually allows for greater or faster gains in speech therapy. Parents would expect academic issues to be helped by tutoring, but often vestibular treatment can lead to ocular-motor improvements that make reading and learning easier and more enjoyable for the child. Many times a caregiver is not all that concerned about a child's clumsiness, because many children are clumsy and grow out of it to some degree. However, when treating the child for the caregiver's primary concern, whatever it may be, the child's motor coordination improves as well.

All sensory and motor skills are connected in a web that creates our reality. Our ability to respond to our environment with accuracy, adapt and learn is a combination of sensory intake and motor output. The result of appropriate treatment and normalization of the vestibular and auditory systems is more accurate sensory intake for a more adaptive motor response; not just splinter skills of rote response and learned behavior. We all want to see our children succeed with as little assistance as possible. When my first child was born, my friend Katie shared with me the secret of successful parenting. She said, "Robin, childhood is a race to independence, and the parent who gets their child there first, wins."

The Specifics of Treatment
In My Clinic

My interaction with a child begins with an evaluation, during which I might perform one or two standardized tests of the child's motor skills; both gross (large) motor skills such as running, and fine motor skills, such as using scissors. While I am looking for areas in which the child may fall behind their peers in skill development, I'm also watching *how* the child approaches different tasks. Knowing that a child can cut out a circle while following the line precisely, but cannot gallop like a horse at age five tells me that, while stationary, his visual-motor skills might be excellent, but his body awareness and vestibular mechanisms allowing for efficient movement need to be addressed through therapy.

The evaluation would also include gathering information from the child's primary caregivers regarding their concerns, the child's preferences and behaviors, and the child's medical history. A parent is a wonderful source of information and a large part of my evaluation is just talking to the parent about how their child makes it through their day. What do they struggle with? What does the parent feel the child should be doing or doing better? What does the child do that the parent feels is dysfunctional? My questions fall into three broad categories: Eating, Sleeping, and Behavior.

1. How is his/her appetite? Does he/she eat a variety of foods? Are mealtimes a problem? Is the parent concerned from the child's nutritional intake?

2. Does the child sleep appropriately for his/her age? What is the bedtime routine like? Is he/she an excessively heavy or light sleeper?

3. How does he/she respond when "things don't go his/her way"? Are schedule changes handled fairly easily? How does

the child behave around his/her siblings? Are there difficulties at school?

This part of the interview opens the floor for the parent to share anything they feel might be helpful to me and anything they are particularly concerned about regarding their child's development and how their child interacts with his/her family, school and friends.

After interacting with the child for however long is possible or necessary to gain some insight into their function, I will recommend therapy or some other course of action. Then the ball falls into the parent's court to decide if therapy will be worth the time and energy expended. One of my jobs during the evaluation is to help the parent understand what I am evaluating, how their child's internal systems could be inaccurate and therefore affecting his development, and what therapy can do to affect that situation. If I decide that the child would benefit from therapy, I will make the case as best I can, conveying as much of the information in the preceding chapters of this book as I feel I can at the time. But the decision to participate in therapy falls on the child's caregiver; and that is fair because he or she will be doing the better part of the interaction and follow-through to help that child.

Vestibular Treatment: My Essentials

There are certain pieces of equipment or techniques that I consider almost essential to treat any child. Here they are, in no particular order, with explanations on how I use them and why I consider them so important.

- The Astronaut Training© Protocol by Mary Kawar, Sheila Frick and Ron Frick. This is a lovely, organized, sound-based, easy-to-follow, inexpensive protocol of vestibular and ocular-motor exercises that I absolutely take liberties with, depending on the child's needs. But one could use the protocol completely as written, and it would be very effective. The ideas and activities outlined in this short book, along with the instructive music-based CD, make short work of beginning treatment of vestibular and connected ocular-motor issues. It's clear for families to follow as homework, which I often assign for about a month. It has a clearly-delineated sequence of treatment that a parent or novice therapist can easily follow, and an experienced therapist can easily adapt (as I do).

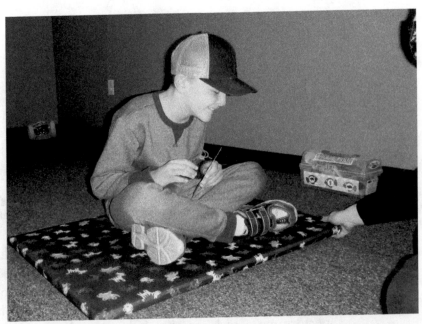

Fig. A-1: Child preparing to rotate on Astronaut Training board.

- A ceiling-mounted swing. I use this tool all the time; to mount a platform swing, a net swing, or a hanging ladder. The tools I use all require different motor responses from a child, from passive tolerance to active holding on, to prediction of movement to interact with me for a game. If the swing is ceiling-mounted, I can achieve levels of movement (in both size and speed) that can "break through" a child's neurologically-established resistance to feeling vestibular input. Itinerant swings, which are suspended from a mobile stand, just don't work as well, I find. As the therapist, I can't safely get a child moving fast or far enough.

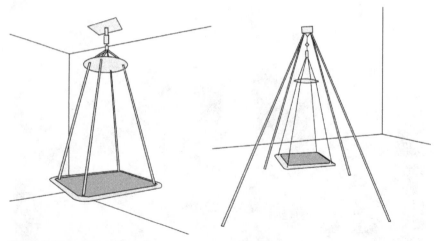

Fig. A-2: The ceiling-mounted swing on the right is preferable to an itinerant swing (left) because it allows for greater arcs of movement and therefore more gravitational force.

- A mobile platform like a mechanical surfboard, wobble board or, to lesser extent, a vibrating platform. This requires a child to balance, react to changes in a surface and perhaps concentrate of performing a task, so that balance and vestibular reactions can be moved to the subconscious part of the brain. Being up on the platform also requires them to be aware of the tipping point of their balance and when they must step off to keep from falling over.

- The remainder of the items I like to have are usually available in any well-outfitted OT or other pediatric clinic. I like to have things that mark the floor, like mobile rubber stepping stones or circles for jumping and stepping activities (think hopscotch). I like stepstools because so much motor planning and balance are involved to use them in sequence. I like to have a series of something on hand (most recently it's been a collection of 5-inch, variously-colored bean-bag frogs) that allow for a variety of creative games that require a child to move and look with big (or small) eye and head movements, like a scavenger hunt.

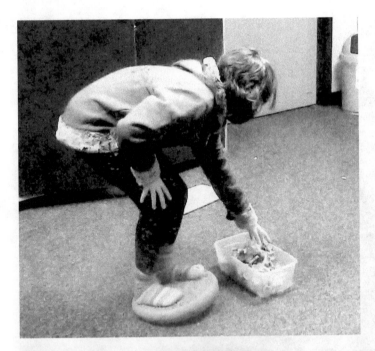

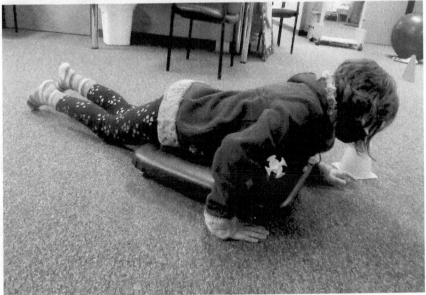

Fig. A-3 (series): Challenging a child's center of gravity and sense of balance.

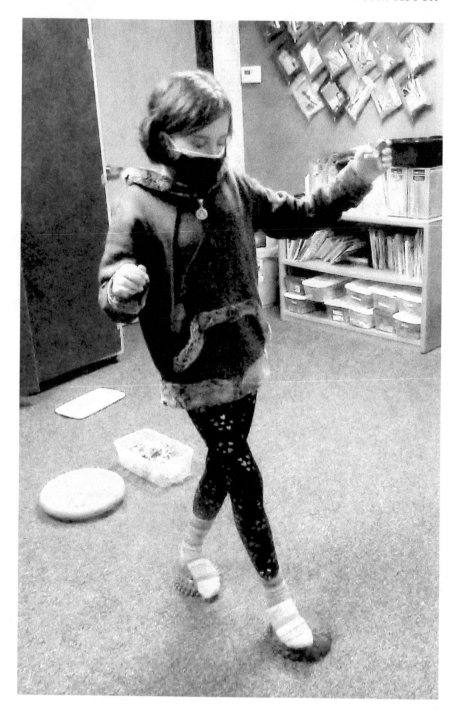

Vestibular therapy in my clinic looks a bit like an indoor playground. Kids move, I move kids, kids move their eyes. I have a sequence and a logic behind the activities we plan. I know vestibular therapy makes an impact because of the results I see, but also because of this occasional scenario; long after a child has been discharged from therapy I might happen upon them in the community. I'm fishing for compliments (which never works) when I ask, "what do you remember about coming to see me?" It's not how much fun I am, or the fact that they can do new things—it's all about the swings. They love the swings because the swings made them feel good. It's that simple.

As a general rule, a vestibularly hyposensitive child will need large, strong, or fast movements to establish vestibular awareness, then progress to controlled, repetitive movements (such as the Astronaut Training protocol). The vestibularly hypersensitive child will probably need of a slow buildup of large but calm movements, eventually with lots of big arcs that emphasize the down direction through stronger g-forces, just like when one feels heavier when they take-off in a plane. Both types of children will likely need targeted ocular-motor muscle practice and may also need to have the sensory systems they have come to depend on, their vision or proprioception, limited in some way. The child's response to these choices (fear, laughter, excitement, queasiness) informs my subsequent choices for therapy. I rely on the parent to be my data-collector after the child leaves the clinic. Was a child nauseous later that day? Did the child sleep very well that night? Was the child more communicative or seem more "with it"? All of these bits of information about how a child responds to my intervention help to guide the ensuing choices regarding what the child needs to experience in my clinic.

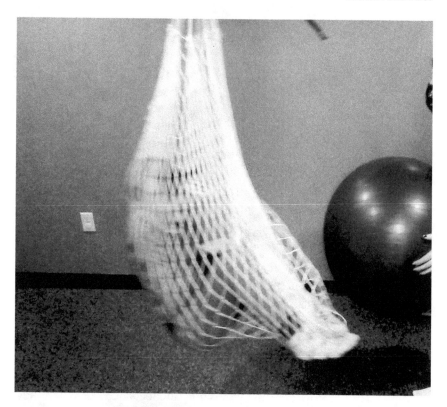

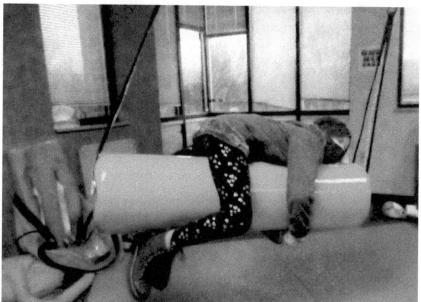

Fig. A-4 (series): Moving the vestibulae in big, new and different ways with swings.

Auditory Treatment: My Essentials

As mentioned in the body of the book, my chosen form of auditory therapy is Therapeutic Listening, which I chose for a variety of reasons. I think it is the most comprehensive, flexible and cost-effective system on the market. But it's certainly not the only choice. Other choices and their characteristics are listed in the chart below. Any therapist you choose should be able to articulate why they chose the system that they use. Please note that the descriptor "Both" indicates that, while some components of the program can be done at home, you will have to contact a certified provider for evaluation and set-up; the indicator "Home" means that the program is available commercially and does not need a professional's intervention (although it is strongly recommended by me).

Different Forms of Auditory Therapy Using Electronically-Modified Sound					
Name of therapy	Clinic vs. Home use	Voice Com-ponent	Spatial Sound Component	Commercial ly Available	Length of Program
Tomatis	Both	Yes	No	No	As Prescribed
SAMONAS	Home	No	Yes	Yes	8 weeks
Auditory Integration Training	Both	No	No	No	As Prescribed
The Listening Program	Home	No	No	No	8 weeks
Therapeutic Listening	Both	No	Yes	No	As Prescribed
Integrated Listening System	Both	Yes	No	Yes	As Prescribed
EASe CDs	Home	No	Yes	Yes	As needed
Binaural Beat	Home	No	No	Yes	As needed

When I opened my own clinic, I bought enough headphones and music chips (at the time the music was stored on SD cards) so that I could give each child I treated a pair of headphones and their prescribed chips for the duration of their time with me. I just didn't have the patience to wait for the child to make progress while only listening during their therapy sessions in the clinic. So, at least theoretically, each child listened to their prescribed chip for a week or two (as their progress went), for 30 minutes, twice a day. Life happens and people are busy. I'd be surprised if any parents were able to stick to that schedule. Maybe some did. But I think they all did what they were capable of, and the vast majority of the time, that was enough.

Different therapy programs have different requirements. Beyond the 60-minutes of listening I prescribed each day, there were a few caveats. No video games or TV while listening. It was a great idea to have a child listen at dinner. They could participate in family conversation if they wished, or just focus on the sounds. They could listen while in the car. They could listen while doing chores or homework. Sometimes a child would need to be in a small space, like a closet while listening and playing quietly. That usually meant a younger sibling was making them uncomfortable in some way during their listening sessions. The family and I worked out the details as we went along.

Adjunct Therapies: What I Like

It would be difficult to enumerate all the potential additional therapies that, when combined with the above approaches, could benefit your child. Instead, here's a short list of my favorites. You can use Google to explore them and see if they seem like something to ask your child's therapist about.

- Kinesiology tape, or some variation thereof, both for its sensory-awareness-building properties and its physical support. One of my favorite applications is to tape a child's *orbicularis oris* muscle around their mouths to support increased midline and oral-motor awareness.

- Wilbarger Deep Pressure and Proprioceptive Technique© (sometimes called the Wilbarger Sensory Therapeutic Brushing Protocol). This is a very specific series of tactile and proprioceptive inputs for a child on a specific schedule, and training should be taken before implementing it.

- The Beckman Oral Motor Program©, particularly her Five-times trials for encouraging a child to try new foods and her mouth exercises for specific muscles.

- Ball-a-vis-x© and The Learning Breakthrough©, which are both higher-level, pre-packaged series of exercises that encourage focus, balance and coordination and come with all the requisite equipment and instructions.

I thought it might be beneficial for you to read about some cases in which these adjunct therapies fit into the broader picture of my therapeutic approach. In the first two cases, therapy went (mostly) according to plan. Each child needed a combination of auditory and vestibular therapy, but with very different goals because they were having very different problems. Harold was as sweet as pie, but his movements were clumsy, he seemed very hyperactive, and his communication skills were lagging. Henry was more in control of his movements than was Harold, but he was not in control of his emotions and behaviors. Lance, Lyndsey and Brent are children who taught me something new. Each of them plateaued during therapy in some specific behavior and that required me to think beyond vestibular and auditory therapy. By adding something new and supportive to the therapy they were receiving, they were able to move to the next level of function.

Case Studies

Harold

When I met Harold, he was an engaging four-year-old with the most adorable head of red curls I'd ever seen. His mother reported that he had always been healthy and was born full-term after a normal pregnancy. Harold lived at home with his parents and older sister. His mother was concerned because Harold was never able to sit still, even for short meals, was rambunctious and clumsy, and wasn't able to produce any of the drawings or crafts that his sister had at his age.

On a standardized motor tests, Harold scored in the "Poor" range for both gross motor and fine motor skills. He seemed to have particular issues holding any physical position, such as standing still with his feet together, or executing any skill that involved moving things around in his hands, such as eating with utensils or holding a crayon. Harold had some minor articulation problems, but his bigger problem while speaking was slowing down and expressing an idea in its entirety. He also needed directions repeated several times before he "heard" them. It seemed that while Harold was on the move, receiving feedback from his joints and muscles, he could be fairly well coordinated. But his coordination was much lower when asked to hold still and his stationary balance was almost non-existent. He was also unable to shift his gaze from one penlight to another or follow my penlight across his field of vision.

Auditorily, Harold had trouble distinguishing individual speech sounds, and thus his speech was difficult to understand. He may have had trouble isolating speech in background noise or trouble processing the meaning behind speech, hence needing directions repeated. He lacked an awareness of the center of his body, which can be enhanced through the bilateral activity of listening. I knew his initial plan of listening must include albums which allowed his stapedius muscle to hear and respond to high and low frequencies with ease, albums with emphasis on emotional content so that he could better understand the meaning behind the words others used, and deep rhythms to enhance his core awareness (think deep bass in dance music, it gets our center moving).

Harold lost his balance when seated on my platform swing, so we began our vestibular therapy with simple movements in the net swing, and spinning on a platform on the floor. Initially, Harold would fall over during seated spinning, because he was unable to depend on the muscles of his legs and body that usually helped him stay upright. *He* wasn't doing the movement, I was spinning the board under him. All that was required of him was to feel the sensations and try to contract the correct muscles to stay upright. As he progressed with these skills, I would add complexity to the games we played to challenge his balance. For example, when we sat together on the floor to play a game, he initially leaned on my lap for support. After a few weeks, I asked him to sit across from me, but he still needed to place his hands on the floor for support. I began to give him cues to take his hands off the floor to depend more on his balance, and he was able to rise to the challenge.

The games we played involved Harold scanning the area around him for game pieces or items I'd requested. Part of the therapy I prescribed for him at home was a regimented plan of vestibular and eye movements. As this therapy progressed, his ability to visually scan the area of the game we were playing increased, and if the game was based on speed, he could even beat me sometimes.

Over the first two months of treatment, Harold's stationary motor control and ocular-motor control developed quite nicely. He could sit for longer amounts of time, and his mother was pleasantly surprised to come into his room at home to find him seated quietly, flipping through a book. That had certainly never happened before. However, when Harold was on the move, his motor control and level of arousal would deteriorate and he would become clumsy and rambunctious. His eye movements were still not well-controlled, and he became visually disoriented while moving around, and therefore slipped back into his old habits of being dependent on his muscles and joints for input.

At this point, it was beneficial to introduce an album into his auditory therapy that involved natural sounds recorded in a spatially-enhanced environment. In his headphones, a bird might sound like it was calling from his right side, behind him, or a cricket might be on the ground in front of him. The idea here was to help his brain better establish the sound-location/eye-movement connection when he *wasn't* wearing the headphones. This seemed to do the trick, and within the next two months, his eye movements were normal.

I was able to discharge Harold from therapy after three-and-a-half months, having met his mother's goals for therapy. He could participate in academic pursuits at an age-appropriate level, sit for a socially-appropriate amount of time, and his movements around his space were more coordinated and much safer.

Henry

Six-year-old Henry's misbehavior in school was such an ongoing problem that he had been assigned a teacher's aide to help manage his behavior. He had trouble with impulse control, rude comments and yelling, and interrupting others. During his evaluation, I noticed that his voice was flat and expressed little emotionality, unless he was angry, as he was when I insisted on handing puzzle pieces to him one at a time from various locations. He had trouble holding any position and could not sit cross-legged without bracing himself with his hands on the floor. He could not move his eyes to follow targets. In attempting to do this, he actually pointed his tongue to the same side as was the visual target; as if to give his brain another cue to know where to move his eyes. He had no post-rotary nystagmus and was hypersensitive to sidelying rotation.

While his flat vocal tone was an indication of a need for auditory therapy, I was more concerned regarding his almost instant anger when asked to look around for puzzle pieces and his hypersensitivity to sidelying rotation. I believed that his brain was processing very little vestibular information. This was affecting his ability to move his eyes around his environment effectively. He was having to use his conscious mind to create motor plans and was not able to adapt quickly to changes. Because his ocular-motor skills were not adequate to see and assess incoming threats, and because he felt so unstable in his body, almost everything was perceived as threat-

ening. For security, he wanted to control his environment as much
as possible. This is not possible during a school day with other
children. Any time he sensed a loss of his control, he felt threatened
and his emotional response was anger. It was as if he was trapped in
a loop of being unpleasantly surprised by just about everything.
Understandably, this made him frustrated and angry as he became
less and less oriented as his day went on. In addition, this heightened sense of aggressive emotions likely made it difficult for him to
feel and express other emotions, such as pleasant surprise or
contentment.

Therapy began with as much intensive movement as he could
tolerate to help him develop the ability to sense movement more
accurately. He was in need of additional input like oral motor
stimulation and deep pressure to help anchor him in space as well.
We began to work on developing his ocular-motor skills, both
through activities and with the help of natural-sounds auditory
therapy.

Progress was slower than I'd expected. At one month, he could
complete all the rotations in the Astronaut Training program, but
could only move his eyes to or follow targets about 3-5 times
consecutively, still making the facial movements to one side or the
other. By the second month his behavior at home, where he had
more control over the environment, had improved and he was
having fewer tantrums. He was able to keep his balance on the platform swing without his hands and he was developing an increased
emotional vocal range. At three months, we could play games in
which he was moving *and* interacting with an object. His ability to
stay with a task, even if the task was frustrating, was much better.
At the discontinuation of therapy, he would complete the majority
of school days without a behavioral incident, was sleeping better,
could concentrate long enough to complete a game or read a book,
and was more flexible in his thoughts. He still had only minimal
post-rotary nystagmus, meaning that his eyes and vestibular system
were not in completely effortless communication. However, for
Henry, that might have meant that he might not be as good at ball-
type games as other children, but he could certainly participate
safely and completely in his entire day, to learn and grow with
friends.

Lance

As a first-born child, Lance's mother was unsure of how much of his behavior was "normal" and how much was due to his complicated birth and early life. He was born during an emergency c-section after his mother developed pre-eclampsia. He was very slow to grow during his early childhood, and also had multiple ear infections and torticollis, a condition in which the head is fixed into rotation to a particular side most of the time.

During his evaluation, I noticed that he had very low balance, walking up steps slowly and needing to place both feet on each step. The normal pattern of movement for an almost-five year-old would be to put one foot on each stair. He had low muscle tone and tripped over the edge of the mats in the room several times. Another clue to his low body and situational awareness was his insistence that he bring toys with him everywhere, one in each hand. The consistent feel of the objects in his hands anchored him during the transition from place to place. I see this behavior often, and I consider it therapeutic progress when a child no longer needs these "anchors."

These clues initially lead me to believe that he was vestibularly-hyposensitive. When treatment began, Lance lost his balance with nearly every activity we attempted and was not able to follow directions well enough to attempt modifications. As we progressed with vestibular therapy, his ocular-motor skills and balance didn't improve as I had expected them to. However, he responded very well to the music of auditory therapy, and he began to process auditory input more quickly. His mother was finding him easier to communicate with and less prone to tantrums. Slowly his balance improved to the point that we could sit together crossed-legged on the floor to play with a toy. He was even able to follow cues to stop using his hands to support his body.

His awareness of his surroundings increased such that he could come into my room, stop at the door, glance around the room and develop a plan for play. He began to be able to hold visual images in his head and recall them with suggestions; so that if his mother said, "It's time to go to school", he could conjure the image of "school" and mentally prepare himself for that environment. Transitions became easier. He seemed more keyed-in to what was happening around him.

One of the areas in which progress was slow for Lance was the development of ocular-motor control. He could scan his environment better within the first few months, but sending his eyes intentionally to locate a specific toy or maintain visual focus on a game was still challenging for him. He was not responding well to the eye exercises that I prescribed. In frustration with our lack of progress, I moved ocular-motor skills to the back burner and changed the focus of treatment to oral motor skills, hoping to address his picky eating and articulation problems more directly. And voila! His ocular-motor skills also improved noticeably.

Lance taught me that some children need to know where the middle of their body is to send their eyes to the right or left. I was also surprised by how much the structure of his face had changed as the muscles began to come alive with movement. As he became more aware of the muscles of his face, and more able to hear the emotional content of others' speech and see the emotion in their face, he began to use those muscles to express his own emotions through his face and voice. He became a more animated child, and the muscles of his face developed to give his face more structure and definition. I have also seen this effect in several of the children with Down Syndrome who I have treated. It's as if their face matures from a baby's to a young child's overnight. It's pretty cool.

Lyndsey

When I met Lyndsey, she was five years old, with a history of multiple ear infections. She was clumsy and ran into things, was always on the go, and unable to sit still to concentrate on any task for more than a few minutes. Her mother reported that she still responded to noises with a startle reflex and could not tolerate a noisy or busy environment like a restaurant or party. But her mother's biggest concern was Lyndsey's lack of variety in her diet. Around 18 months, Lyndsey began gagging and rejecting any new foods, even some foods she had previously eaten. Her mother described her diet as "beige", consisting of grilled cheese sandwiches and pasta. She had a few food allergies, but was avoiding foods her mother knew to be safe as well.

During my evaluation, I determined that Lyndsey had ocular-motor issues, sound-localization problems and decreased vestibular awareness. It turned out she was one of those tricky kids who initially appear vestibularly-hyposensitive. Over the course of two months of therapy, her sustained attention improved markedly, her sleep became better and more regular (a problem her mother didn't share with me at her initial evaluation because she didn't believe anything could be done about it), and her behavior matured into that of a typical of a five-year-old. While Lyndsey was more willing to try new foods, mealtimes still involved a lot of gagging, arguments, and some histrionics on Lyndsey's part. She had improved so much in the past couple months in every other area, what was happening with eating? Were Lyndsey and her family just reacting out of habits they had built over the years? Over the next month, her mother and I problem-solved **mealtime behaviors** from a habit-pattern perspective, analyzing how the high emotion level of mealtimes could be brought down and how to respond to negative behavior. The family made the following changes:

1. Mealtimes could last no more than 20 minutes, with a timer set at the beginning of the meal. When the timer went off, the food was removed from the table. If Lyndsey had spent her mealtime having a tantrum, then she missed out on dinner.

2. No one was allowed to make negative comments about the food, just as a child is taught not to say rude things when visiting a friend's house for dinner. Lyndsey's parents were not allowed to discuss her intake at the table, and discussion was only to be quiet family sharing.

3. Before dinner, Lyndsey's mom set up TV trays in the living room as an alternate eating location. Lyndsey was told that she could refuse food if she wanted to, but if she threw a tantrum over what was on her plate, the family would retreat to the living room to eat in peace. This was not intended to be a punishment and was carried out with no commentary and a neutral tone.

Over that month, Lyndsey's social behaviors continued to improve and mealtimes began to quiet down. Eventually, Lyndsey got hungry enough at mealtimes to try new foods calmly and decide whether or not she liked them. Family meals became enjoyable and Lyndsey found she could tolerate many of the foods she dreaded.

Brent

Sometimes a child makes wonderful progress, but doesn't realize that they are more coordinated, more communicative, and more engaged with the world around them. They just know that they feel better, but don't necessarily know that their ability to tolerate new things has changed. Perhaps that is why they continue with old habit patterns when it comes to eating. Brent was one such case. When I met him, he was a large-for-his-age 10 year old boy who moved very rigidly. His mother reported that he had 7-8 ear infections every year as a child until pressure-equalization tubes were placed in his ear drums. He had no friends at school and preferred to stay in his room, making elaborate Lego creations. He could only converse on a narrow range of topics and didn't seem to listen to others. He had little vocal range or facial expression, and he was a very picky eater.

His evaluation revealed that he was extremely vestibularly *and* auditorily hypersensitive, and he preferred to be stationary and use his eyes to orient himself in space. After two months of treatment, he had big improvements in movement, communication and sleep. After three months, he was playing outside with his dad more often, was connecting with others at school, and his teachers were noticing how much more mobile and social he was. However, there was very limited progress involving eating. His mother had begun to work with him on making smoothies in the kitchen to increase his fruit and vegetable consumption. But she was too often met with resistance and an insistence that he "didn't like that food" at mealtimes. I knew he had made the neurological changes necessary to broaden his palette without gagging, but the memory of that discomfort was keeping him from trying things.

So we instituted "eating practice." These are times outside of meals when he could work on the requirements of eating without the pressure of his family worrying about him skipping a meal or missing nutrients. He and I worked together in the clinic using Beckman's Target Food Worksheet, in which Brent needed to look at the food five times, touch it five times, kiss it five times, etc. He worked his way up to five full bites, knowing we would stop if he gagged or couldn't tolerate the next progression. And he was welcome to spit the food out if he was able to take a bite, but not to swallow it. In this way we tackled apples, peas, eggs, and a few other foods. His homework was to continue the practice with the same foods until we met again. However, he became bored between sessions and would use the 5-Times to try a new food, usually breezing through the trials but needing a little time on the chewing and swallowing phases. Most importantly, he learned that something he has not liked or had not been able to tolerate in the past might not always be that way. That type of mental flexibility will serve him well as he continues to encounter new situations and learn new things throughout his life.

Glossary

Amygdala: Area within each half of the brain (pl. Amygdalae), part of the limbic system with which the brain processes emotions.

Auditory System: The pinna, eardrum, bones of the middle ear, cochlea, nerves running from the ear to the brain, and associated brain centers involved in sensing, interpreting and responding to sounds in the environment.

Body Scheme: Innate understanding on one's body parts, their relationship to one another, and their position in space.

Cochlea (pl. Cochleae): Snail-shaped organ of the inner ear, that contains membranes and small hair-like cells stimulated by specific frequencies of air waves, that allow the brain to receive sounds.

Dorsal Columnar Nucleus (DCN): Structure of the brainstem that processes fine touch and proprioceptive information from the body, but is also one of the first locations to which a neural impulse from the ear travels.

Echolalia: Common behavior in people with autism in which they repeat words or phrases, either what has been recently said to them or that they have heard in the past, with no perceptible attempt to communicate.

Echolocation: The ability to locate an object via listening, either by sound emitted from it or from sounds reflecting off it. Notably used by dolphins, bats and birds to locate prey and predators, but humans have nascent echolocation abilities as well.

Efferent Nerves: Nerves running from the brain and central nervous system to sensory organs and muscles for both voluntary and involuntary motor control

Extraocular Muscles: Six muscles that control the direction of the eye orb within its socket, controlled by cranial nerves.

Feedforward: Complex system of vestibular, muscle and neural awareness that allows us to subconsciously calculate physical effects on our bodies and objects around us. Example, feedforward allows us to predict how much force is required to open a door or allows us to catch an object that has been knocked off a table before it hits the floor. Feedforward allows us to react to what is in the process of happening.

Gravitational Insecurity: Fearful reaction to movement which is not within one's control or involves one's feet being off the ground or one's head being out of an upright position.

Habituation: Decreased notice of or response to a stimulus that is presented repeatedly.

Harmonics: Superimposed sound waves that, taken as a whole, make for a specific sound pitch, but may create a unique timbre. For example, an oboe and a flute both playing middle C will sound different to the ear because they have different harmonic tones.

Hippocampus (pl. hippocampi): Neural structure within each lobe of the brain essential to the formation of memories.

Lateral Superior Olive (LSO): A structure of the midbrain responsible for comparison of sound intensity between ears, playing a role in sound localization.

Medial Superior Olive (MSO): A structure of the brainstem that measures differences between ears related to the timing of sound's arrival to the ear, playing a role in sound localization.

Mismatch Negativity (MMN): Measurable component of electrical activity in the brain when an unusual or unexpected auditory stimulus is presented, e.g. an new or unrecognizable sound within the environment, such as a dog barking in the delivery ward of a hospital.

Neural Plasticity: The capacity of the brain and neural system to create new connections with repeated activity, or to prune unused connections.

Neurodiverse: Blanket term for people on the spectrum of autism, with attention-deficit hyperactivity disorder or sensory-processing disorder.

Neurotypical: Term used to refer to people not displaying autistic-like or unusual behavior. Used to avoid using the term "normal", as people with autism are not "abnormal" or "wrong" and "normal" is a very poorly-defined construct.

Nystagmus: Involuntary movement of the eyes across the visual field.

Orienting Response: A behavioral response to a novel stimulus. The beginning of the chain of reactions necessary to answer the questions "what is this new thing?" and "is this new thing a threat?"

Pinna: The external ear.

Pitch Relativity: The relationship of vocal tone from one moment to the next, a larger change in tone indicating a more emotion-ally-charged communication; e.g., the sudden rise in vocal pitch when one begins to talk about a subject they find exciting.

Proprioceptive: Relating to internal sensation regarding position of body parts, relative to other body parts; e.g., knowing your arm has lifted away from your torso without having to confirm it visually.

Reticular Formation: Interconnected centers within the brainstem that regulate incoming sensory information and help the brain modulate it's level of alertness appropriately.

Reticular Activating System (RAS): Part of the reticular formation that influences states of sleep or wakefulness by modulating sensory and motor information between the brain and body.

Sensory Integration Treatment: Therapy developed by A. Jean Ayres to address emotional dysregulation, behavioral and learning issues exhibited by children with sensory processing disorder (SPD).

Sound Database: Catalog of neural patterns stored in the cerebral cortex that are related to repeated or common sounds or speech patterns.

Sound Localization: The neurological ability to locate the source of a sound within the environment.

Spectral Qualities: Grouping of sound characteristics that allow the brain to categorize and predict sounds, e.g., all woodwind instruments sound similar (but not the same) when playing the same pitch, and the brain will group the sound with like sounds based on harmonic overtone and intensity of sound.

Stapedius: Small muscle in either inner ear that dampens vibration of the stapes bone, thus allowing modulation of incoming frequencies of sounds and allowing the ear to "focus" on the sounds the brain would like to hear more clearly.

Stimulus-specific Adaptation (SSA): The neurological process that allows for habituation, a dampening impulse sent to a specific sensory system to limit the flow of incoming sensory stimuli.

Tensor Tympani: Small muscles in either inner ear connected to the malleus bone and thus to the eardrum. When the tensor tympani contracts, it limits the intensity of vibration of the eardrum and protects our hearing from overly-loud sounds, including our own voice as conducted through the bones and tissues of our body.

Vestibular System: Sensory system responsible for informing the brain and body regarding self- and other-generated movement, body and head position, and helping to create a spatial map within the brain for navigation. Provides information regarding body position for posture maintenance, movement for the planning of physical interactions, and physical stability to allow for the division of attention.

Vestibulum (pl. Vestibulae): Sensory end organs that sense the position and movement of the head in gravity-bound space.

Working Memory: A cognitive system that allow for short-term storage and retrieval of information to allow for contiguous thought and task completion.

Index of Behaviors

References

Ayres, A.J. (2005). *Sensory Integration and the Child* (25th Anniversary Edition). Western Psychological Services.

Angelaki, D.E. & Cullen, K.E. (2008). Vestibular system: The many facets of a multimodal sense. *Annual Review of Neuroscience, 31,* 125-150.

Antoine, M.W., Vijayakumar, S., McKeehan, N., Jones, S.M., & Herbert, J.M. (2017). The severity of vestibular dysfunctionin deafness as a determinant of comorbid hyperactivity or anxiety. *Journal of Neuroscience, 37*(20), 5144-5154.

Antoine, M.W., Hubner, C.A., Arezzo, J.C., & Hebert, J.M. (2013). A causative link between inner ear defects and long-term striatal dysfunction. *Science, 341*(6150), 1120-1123.

Bajo, V.M., Nodal, F.R., Moore, D.R., & King, A.J. (2010). The descending corticocollicular pathway mediates learning-induced auditory plasticity. *Nature Neuroscience 13*(2), 253-262.

Baranek, M. & Lambert, F.M. (2009). Impaired perception of gravity leads to altered head direction signals: What can we learn from vestibularly-deficient mice? *Journal of Neurophysiology, 102,* 12-14.

Barry, S.R. (2009). *Fixing My Gaze: A scientist's journey into seeing in three dimensions.* Basic Books.

Bennett, K.E., Haggard, M.P., Silva, P.A. & Stewart, I.A. (2001). Behavioural and developmental effects of otitis media with effusion into the teens. *Archives of Disease in Childhood, 85,* 91-95.

Berger, D.S. (2016). Eurythmics for Autism and Other Neurophysiologic Diagnoses: A sensorimotor music-based approach. Jessica Kingsley.

Bertleson, P. & Radeau, M. (1981). Cross-modal bias and perceptual fusion with auditory-visual spatial discordance. *Perception and Psychophysics, 29*(6), 578-584.

Biel, L. & Peske, N. (2018). *Raising a Sensory Smart Child: The definitive handbook for helping your child with sensory integration issues* (updated edition). Penguin.

Borg, E. & Counter, S.A. (1989). The middle ear muscles. *Scientific American, 261*(2), 74-81.

Clark, D.L. (2009). The vestibular system: An overview of structure and function. In K.J. Ottenbacher & M.A. Short-DeGraff (Eds.), *Vestibular Processing Dysfunction in Children* (pp. 5-32). Hawthorn Press.

Condon, W.S. (1975). Multiple response to sound in dysfunctional children. *Journal of Autism and Childhood Schizophrenia, 5*(1), 37-56.

Davis, D.S. (2013). *Sound Bodies Through Sound Therapy, electronic edition.* Sound Words Ink.

Davis, D.S. (2016). *The Cycle of Sound: A Missing Energetic Link* (2nd edition). Sound Words Ink.

Day, B.L. & Fitzpatrick, R.C. (2005). The vestibular system. *Current Biology, 15*(15), 583-586.

Frick, S.M. & Young, S.R. (2009). *Listening With the Whole Body: Clinical concepts and treatment guidelines for Therapeutic Listening®.* Vital Links.

Gopnik, A., Meltzoff, A.N., & Kuhl, P.K. (2001). *The Scientist in the Crib: What early learning tells us about the mind.* Perennial.

Grandin, T. (2006). *Thinking in Pictures: My life with autism* (2nd edition). Vintage Books.

Heffner, R.S. & Heffner, H.E. (1992). Visual factors in sound localization in mammals. *Journal of Comparative Neurology, 317*(3), 219-232.

Higashida, N. (2016). *The Reason I Jump: The inner voice of a thirteen-year-old boy with autism* (2nd edition, K.A. Yoshida and D. Mitchell, Trans.). Random House.

Hitier, M., Besnard, S., & Smith, P.F. (2014). Vestibular pathways involved in cognition. *Frontiers in Integrative Neuroscience, 8*, 1-16.

Hopson, J.L. (1998). Fetal psychology. *Psychology Today, 31*(5), 44-48.

Jacewicz, N. (2015, December 7). *Inside the mind of a picky eater.* The Atlantic. https://www.theatlantic.com/health/archive/2015/12/psychology-picky-eating-kids/418959/

Joliffe, T, Lansdown, R, & Robinson, C. (1992). Autism: A personal account. *Communication, 26*, 12-19.

Klass, P. & Costello, E. (2021). *Quirky Kids: Understanding and supporting your child with developmental differences* (updated edition). American Academy of Pediatrics.

Madaule, P. (2015). *When Listening Comes Alive: A guide to effective learning and communication* (Revised Electronic Edition). Publish Green. https://www.amazon.com/When-Listening-Comes-Alive-Madaule-ebook/dp/B00TU609MY/

Mailloux, Z., Leão, M., Becerra, T.A., Mori, A.B., Soechting, E., Roley, S.S., Buss, N., & Cermak, S.A. (2014). Modification of the postrotary nystagmus test for evaluating young children. *American Journal of Occupational Therapy, 68*, 514-521.

Maurer, D. & Maurer, C. (1988). *The World of the Newborn.* Basic Books.

Meng, H, May P.J., Dickman, D., & Angelaki, D.E. (2007). Vestibular signals in primate thalamus: properties and origins. *Journal of Neuroscience, 27*(50), 13590-13602.

Miller, L.J. (2014). *Sensational Kids: Hope and help for children with sensory processing disorder* (revised edition). Perigee.

Moore, J.K. & Linthicum, F.H. (2007). The human auditory system: A timeline of development. *International Journal of Audiology, 46*(9), 460-478.

Nahum, M., Nelken, I., & Ahissar, M. (2008). Low-level information and high-level perception: The case of speech in noise. *PLoS Biology, 6*(5), 1-14.

Nelken, I. & Ahissar, M. (2006). High-level and low-level processing in the auditory system: the role of the primary auditory cortex. In P. Divenyi, S. Greenberg, & G. Meyer (Eds.), *Dynamics of Speech Production and Perception* (pp. 343-354). IOS Press.

Oetter, P, Richter, E.W., & Frick, S.M. (1995). *M.O.R.E.: Integrating the mouth with sensory and postural functions* (2nd edition). Pileated Press.

Paavelainen, P., Arajärvi, P., & Takegata, R. (2007). Preattentive detection of nonsalient contingencies between auditory features. *Neuroreport, 18*(2), 159-163.

Patel, A. (2015). *Music and the Brain: Course guidebook.* The Great Courses.

Polley, D.B., Steinberg, E.E., & Merzenich, M.M. (2006). Perceptual learning directs auditory cortical map reorganization through top-down influences. *Journal of Neuroscience, 26*(18), 4970-4982.

Pressnitzer, D., Sayles, M., Micheyl, C., & Winter, I.M. (2008). Perceptual organization of sound begins in the auditory periphery. *Current Biology, 18,* 1124-1128.

Robinson, C.W. & Sloutsky, V.M. (2007). Visual processing speed: Effects of auditory input on visual processing. *Developmental Science, 10*(6), 734-740.

Reynolds, S., Lane, S.J., & Thacker, L. (2012). Sensory processing, physiological stress, and sleep behaviors in children with and without autism spectrum disorders. *OTJR: Occupation, Participation and Health, 32*(1), 246-257.

Ronca, A.E., Fritzsch, B., Bruce, L.L., & Alberts, J.R. (2008). Orbital spaceflight during pregnancy shapes function of mammalian vestibular system. *Behavioral Neuroscience, 122*(1), 224-232.

Schnupp, J., Nelken, I., & King, A. (2012). *Auditory Neuroscience: Making sense of sound.* MIT Press.

Shah, P. (Executive Producer). (2015-present). Hidden Brain [audio podcast]. National Public Radio. https://www.npr.org/2018/05/14/610796636/baby-talk-decoding-the-secret-language-of-babies.

Shahidullah, S. & Hepper, P.G. (1994). Frequency discrimination by the fetus. *Early Human Development, 36*(1), 13-26.

Shelton, B.R. & Searle, C.L. (1980). The influence of vision on the absolute identification of sound-source position. *Perception & Psychophysics, 28*(6), 589-596.

Thomason, R.T. & Hopper, R. (1992). Pauses, transition relevance, and speaker change. *Human Communication Research, 18*(3), 429-444.

van der Kolk, B.A. (2014). *The Body Keeps the Score: Brain, mind and body in the healing of trauma.* Penguin.

Weiss, M.D., Baer, S., Allan, B.A., Saran, K., & Schibuk, H. (2011). The screens culture: Impact on ADHD. *ADHD Attention Deficit and Hyperactivity Disorders, 3*(4), 327-334.

Williamson, G.G. & Anzalone, M.E. (2001). *Sensory Integration and Self-Regulation in Infants and Toddlers.* Zero-to-Three.

Winkler, I., Háden, G.P., Ladinig, O., Sziller, I., & Honing, H. (2009). Newborn infants detect the beat in music. *Proceedings of the National Academy of Sciences, 106*(7), 2468-2471.

Wittman, M. (2016). *Felt Time: The psychology of how we perceive time* (E. Butler, Trans.). MIT Press.

Yoon, K.H., Köver, H., Insanally, M.N., Semerdjian, J.H., & Bao, S. (2007). Early experience impairs perceptual discrimination. *Nature Neuroscience, 10*(9), 1191-1197.

About the Author

Robin Abbott has been an occupational therapist for over 20 years. She did not learn about the benefits of auditory and controlled vestibular therapy during either her Bachelor's or Master's degree training in occupational therapy. After post-professional training in advanced Therapeutic Listening© and Astronaut Training©, having seen some of the therapy-accelerating effects of these treatments, she was curious about why these treatments were so uniquely powerful. 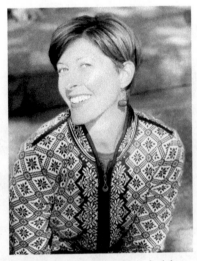 She began cobbling together the available research in her field, as well as neuroscience, audiology and rehabilitation science, creating a more objective picture of the effect of this therapy that confirmed the wonderful improvements she was seeing in her clients.

As she practiced with children throughout the country (having moved a variety of places with her military spouse, Chris) she realized that these effective therapies were not commonly practiced. Historically, other effective treatments have not become widely available without the active involvement of parents, educators, and clinic-based therapists; all of whom insist on the availability of therapy that will help the children they care about. Auditory and controlled-vestibular therapy needed this type of grass-roots push! This book is Robin's effort to inform and enlighten the child-caring community about this treatment, so that they can be the best advocates for their children.

Robin has presented these ideas to parents, therapists and students throughout the US and internationally. She has a TedX talk available online and is the founder of Dovetail Therapy. Now retired, she lives in Iowa with Chris. Still involved in healing, she is a practicing massage therapist and yoga teacher. She has two grown children and enjoys backpacking, reading, and gardening. Visit her online at http://www.booksoundadvice.com/

Index

CPSIA information can be obtained
at www.ICGtesting.com
Printed in the USA
JSHW010051230722
28442JS00001B/1